Alimentary
my dear doctor

With the compliments of

Janis Beaton Duphar Labs

Dec 1988

Medical Anecdotes and Humour

Alimentary
my dear doctor

Edited by Clifford Hawkins

from contributions submitted by members of
the General Practitioner Writers Association

Radcliffe Medical Press · Oxford

© 1988 Radcliffe Medical Press Ltd
27 Park End Street, Oxford OX1 1HU

British Library Cataloguing in Publication Data
Alimentary, my dear doctor.
(Medical anecdotes and humour).
1. Humour in English, 1945–. Special
subjects: Man. Health – Anthologies
I. Hawkins, Clifford   II. Series
827'.914'080355

ISBN 1-870905-05-9

Designed by Oxprint, Oxford
Photoset by Enset, Midsomer Norton, Avon
Printed and bound by Billings, Worcester

Contents

Foreword

The General Practitioner Writers Association is a remarkable phenomenon. It began when two examiners for the membership of the Royal College of General Practitioners met in a bar in the Lake District when attending a course. Both were enthusiastic writers with many publications and inevitably they talked of writing and the fun they derived from it. When the work of the course parted them they agreed that a forum was needed where they and other authors could meet to talk their peculiar brand of shop. Medicine has always spawned writers; think of Conan Doyle, Somerset Maugham, A.J. Cronin, Frances Brett Young, Rowan Williams . . . the list is long and meritorious. For all those known successful names there must be many others in the past whose names never reached fame but who, nevertheless, wrote for their own and others' enjoyment and profit. A browse through the many publications which nowadays thump onto the doctor's doormat shows how many of our colleagues write today. Their subjects too are infinitely varied; some write research papers or review articles, some write plays, novels or poetry. The man or woman who can express thoughts clearly enough to entertain or to create verse has much to teach those of us who essay to write clear medical English.

That idea, conceived over Lakeland bitter, seemed destined for stillbirth, because scores of letters written to likely funding bodies produced polite interest but no material support. It was the Editor of the *Lancet* who really launched the Association. When he heard of the idea an invitation was issued from Adam Square which provided the necessary impetus for the Association to take off. Now, three years later, nearly three hundred authors who write for, from or about general practice from as far afield as Europe, Australasia and the New World have joined the Association. There is a thriving journal under the editorship of one of the original Lakeland pair. Every year there are two workshop meetings where many aspects of the wordsmith's trade are debated and the work of members subjected to kindly constructive criticism. There is a register of members and their particular interests which is circulated to editors and publishers. This has led to a large number of authors receiving commissions for their work. When Radcliffe Medical Press offered a prize for humorous writing the committee of the Association was delighted but a little concerned that perhaps the idea would not fire the membership. This book shows just how wrong they were.

Doctors make good raconteurs and, with their ringside view of other people's lives, always have a cornucopia of anecdotes. This volume is the result of a competition to produce the best short incident and longer tale on the subject of The Guts of General Practice. Despite the committee's hesitation at the enthusiasm of the membership, entries poured in to tease the judgement of the adjudicator, Clifford Hawkins. This sage physician, well known for his penmanship and books on writing and speaking in medicine, is rumoured to have selected only those entries which made him laugh aloud. So we hope that other readers will take similar pleasure in these contributions.

At a time when there is much doubt and uncertainty in the National Health Service and consequential despondency within the profession it is refreshing to see the enthusiasm of this growing group of medical writers who either so enjoy their work that the sheer pleasure of it bursts through or cannot contain their mirth at some of the more ridiculous aspects of human behaviour, be it from patients or the professionals.

ROBIN HULL
General Practitioner Writers Association

Preface

A wealth of material provided by the writers' competition has made it possible to produce a book of original humour rather than an anthology of hackneyed jokes. Forty-one contributions were selected from the sixty-four entries on matters concerned with the digestive system.

Editing and compiling the book has been made easier by the high standard of writing; in fact, not one example of gobbledygook was found. Most contributions contained themes that could be grouped under definite headings, so I have written introductory and link passages to make it a book which can be read from the start to finish; these modest contributions are printed in italics. Anyone dealing with patients – from doctors to paramedical workers and medical students – may, I hope, find that these efforts have been worth while; and the occasional medical term should not confuse the lay reader.

Doctors occupy a front seat at life's stage. Much is tragedy, yet episodes of comedy occur: these, apart from being a welcome relief to doctors, often provide unique examples of humour. Humour should have a background of seriousness to create the incongruity which is its mainspring, and this setting is provided by the nature of a doctor's work. There are many types of humour: the comic, unexpected comparisons, sudden deflation, nonsense, satire and the humour of language – misprints, wrong words, puns and malapropisms. Examples of many of these will be found in the book. A sense of humour is an asset for it puts problems into perspective. Laughter acts as a cathartic and causes relaxation. Such tension relief is an invaluable antidote to the stresses of modern life.

Cartoons were drawn by Dr John Moll. Andrew Bax, the publisher, organised this competition and I am especially grateful to him for his enthusiasm and help, and for his achievement in publishing the book so quickly.

CLIFFORD HAWKINS

Postgraduate Medical Centre,
Queen Elizabeth Hospital,
Birmingham B15 2TQ

To the long-suffering patients without whom this book could not have been written.

1
Introduction

The subject of this book – as perspicacious readers may have dis-covered – concerns the alimentary tract, the title being a pun on Sherlock Holmes' cliché 'Elementary, My Dear Watson'. Innards or guts are colloquial terms and the first writer discusses the curious con-notation of guts with courage and determination.

The Guts of General Practice

So often, the trouble with the English language is under-standing what is meant. What about the 'guts' needed to be a GP? That is, the pluck or determination, fortitude, or even bravery (*OED*) that is required for the daily round. How is it that 'guts' implies such qualities? It was probably Shakespeare who started it when he described 'the bowels' to be 'the seat of the emotions'. Mind you, he didn't have much knowledge of physiology, and he certainly had not met poor Alexis St Martin,* who had his innermost thoughts paraded on view, cour-tesy of his abdominal wound. His gastric lining suffused with rage when his face looked thunderous, but there was little evi-dence of it smiling when he was happy. As far as I know, no changes were recorded when he felt determined or 'strong'.

Is there, then, a courage centre lower down that we call upon when we are girding ourselves for some trial or tribula-tion? It is usually our loins that are called into action on these

---

*Alexis St Martin – in case readers are not aware – was a Canadian youth of 18 who shot himself accidentally when trapping; the powder and shot blew away part of the abdominal wall and perforated the cardiac portion of his stomach. The local surgeon Dr William Beaumont considered the prognosis hopeless but he survived and became the surgeon's servant. Beaumont wrote 'I can look directly into the cavity of the stomach, observe its motion and almost see the process of digestion'. His book *Experiments and Observations on the Gastric Juice and the Physiology of Digestion*, published in 1833, formed the basis of modern physiology of the stomach.

occasions, although I am not sure exactly what this means, either. Are we supposed to put on a kidney belt as in days of old in the tropics, or a jockstrap? While the latter might make one feel more together, as it were, it isn't likely to lift the spirit much, and my recollection is that one was little protected from anything by donning one.

If we take a quick tour through our GI tract, it is difficult to find any organ, with the possible exception of the stomach, which would be, in terms of the words we use, the site of intestinal fortitude. In fact, most of the word associations are relative to darker emotions or worse. Why 'having the stomach' for something is considered to be virtuous, I am not sure either. Surely it means only that one isn't liable to heave at the merest sight of water, or that one wasn't going to throw up all over the dissecting room at the first sight of some undignified human remains? Is one, I wonder, more likely to faint, or tremble, after a partial gastrectomy? A tube gastroplasty is certainly supposed to reduce the stomach and aid slimming, but does it also diminish our 'guts'?

We have missed the tongue, you might say, but not much good comes from it, really. Anything sweet or reasonable really comes from the vocal cords, but if the reverse, the organ is described as 'waspish', or wagging all the time. The emotional responses of the recipient to the latter are usually predictable, but highly unlikely to be uplifting!

The duodenum could be considered next, but in fact only bad vibes emanate from here. More an anxiety centre than anything else, as witnessed by the multimillions spent by drug companies, and then the public, in beating its ulcer into submission. The loins are certainly not girded here. Passing right along, then, we see on our left (or the right, depending on whether you are the operator or operatee) the spleen. The spleen was considered by the Ancients to be the real seat of all emotion, but all we do now is to vent it when we are angry. It can be described as waxy or lardaceous and it is occasionally accused of wandering off, but it never calls us to 'derring do'. It actually gets smaller, if fight or fright are in the offing. If, indeed, it ever gets bigger, that usually means trouble for the owner. By just being there, it causes problems for surgeons.

The bloody thing is always in the way, and seems to have a propensity for bleeding without even being touched. Maybe venting it produces anger, rather than the other way round.

The liver isn't much better, either. Our forbears coupled it with the brain, and called them vital organs. They supposed it to be the seat of love and passion, but 'white-livered' ('lily-' if you are American) now denotes cowardice — 'How manie cowards ... who inwarde searcht have lyeurs white as milke'. Shakespeare again. Hiding just below, although sometimes hanging down lower, to confuse the unwary who confidently diagnose appendicitis, is the gallbladder. The repository of 'black bile and ingratitude' exclaimed one of the fathers of surgery, or was it bile and black ingratitude? No matter, the feeling imparted is the same. Again, the Ancients had kept their physiology simple. A pity, you might say, that it did not stay that way. A former anatomy tutor of mine used to delight in telling us that Morgagni, in his day at Padua, was the Professor both of Anatomy *and* Physiology, and he wrote a textbook combining the then knowledge of the two subjects. It was 'that thick' (separating his fingers by about 1½ inches), 'and,' he said, 'if the physiologists nowadays would confine themselves to what they know, instead of what they think they know, the book would still be no bigger.' Anatomical chauvinism, maybe, but it would certainly make the Primary FRCS examination more passable.

In those days, four 'humours' ran the whole show. There were Blood and Phlegm, who both sound fairly uplifting, and then Cholera, and even worse, Melancholer, or in English, Black Bile. There is not much fortitude, or bravery, here. Irritability or anger come straight out of these last two essences to fire our emotions. The use of the word Cholera would also suggest that these feelings can emerge through the anal canal, and for those who have had it that is a pretty accurate description of the truth. Quite nearby enough to be confusing is the pancreas. I suppose it does actually do something for our guts, since the absence of one of its essential juices produces the most disgusting result. A favourite insult of another of my mentors was to describe the object of his derision (usually one of my fellow students) as a 'pancreatic stool', i.e., bulky, pale, slimy and very offensive-smelling. He did not enlarge on the associated ability to float on water, though. An excess or lack of this organ's hormonal secretions imbalances our blood sugar levels and causes diabetes, but does not directly influence our emotions, although sweetbreads may be soul food to some.

The jejunum is next, but is so-called because it is always seen to be empty after death, and, indeed, it rarely contains much when inspected intra-operatively unless obstructed, so there goes a large part of our 22 feet of tubing as a stirrer of emotions. Our colons are usually filled, but not with fortitude, or determination. The sigmoid is so-called for its S-shape, which it is, and the rectum is supposed to be straight, but it is not, and it ends in the anus, which is just a ring.

In the end, after this brief tour through our guts, there appears to be no obvious place in which resides the source of the emotion that implies courage. Maybe having the guts for something really means having the heart for it.

JOHN TAYLOR
Lichfield

Why The Digestive System?

The Digestive System, as is known by everyone with a medical degree or access to the Reader's Digest *Home Doctor* (much the same thing, if my patients are to be believed), begins at the mouth and ends at er, another place. The Ancients thought the digestive tract was the seat of our emotions, and that its workings were intimately connected with ebbs and flows of the various human passions; hence the identification of acid reflux symptoms with emotional over-indulgence. Come to think of it, perhaps the idea is not so far-fetched. Consider the emetic effect of most television soap operas. Personally, I believe that heartburn is the pain you get in your wallet when you have wined and dined too well and begin to realise that the bill is going to be of the arm and leg variety.

The upper or proximal orifice opens in the middle of the lower face and functions along the lines of a vacuum cleaner. Victuals, licenced or otherwise, are entered more or less at random and commence a remarkable journey, through acid bath and enzyme fields, to be squeezed and griped by fearsome peristalsis waves, only to arrive at journey's end as exhausted and dehydrated as an airline traveller and to be treated in much the same way. The digestive tract is not what you could call 'the scenic route', being smelly, noisy and dark (unless some demented doctor has his fibre-optic telescope up it or down it).

The bottom or distal end is also not generally reckoned to be a pretty sight but, I am led to believe, this view partly depends on your orientation, as the bishop said to the actor.

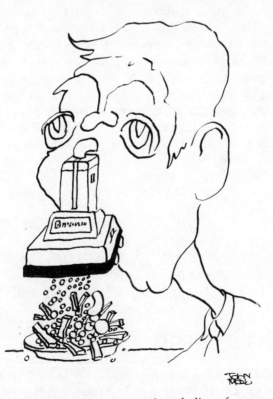

The upper or proximal orifice functions along the lines of a vacuum cleaner

The question which leaps to mind is: 'What is it all for?' Surely it cannot be there simply to keep manufacturers of exotic medical devices in business or to keep gastroenterology departments in employment. But equally, if the Digestive System did not exist, what would be the need for the afore-mentioned items? I believe there are only two possible explanations.

The first possibility is that the Digestive System is a par-ticularly tasteless divine joke. The Almighty could easily have concluded that the best way to keep a sense of frailty and vul-nerability in us humans would be to design us around a long, complex and convoluted tube. The tube would be subject to numerous and inexplicable ailments and be prone to the emis-sion of smells and noises, unpredictable and unstoppable, pre-ferably at the most awkward and socially embarrassing moments. There can be few actions guaranteed to produce a stunned, and possibly respectful, silence during a garden party at Buckingham Palace than the unexpected and un-bridled emission of a Royal burp. Or worse. Apparently, an answering guffaw or titter is not considered Good Form.

The other possibility is that over millenia of evolution the higher animals have developed a most wonderful mechanism for digesting all sorts of food with great efficiency and the minimum of waste.

R. WYNDHAM
Norwich

The following is an allegory of the First World War, written to illus-trate the problems facing a GP. (FPC, Family Practitioner Committee; DN, District Nurse; HV, Health Visitor; BMH, Base Military Hos-pital).

Not Quite Goodbye to All That

It was raining hard, for the fourth day in succession. All around the trench the ground had turned to cloying mud.

'Lots of small arms fire this morning, sir,' the subaltern

shouted to his CO. The CO grunted. He'd seen it all before. 'Any sign of the Major, Perkins?' he asked. 'No, sir. He's on leave, actually.' 'Huh! Short-staffed again, are we?' Perkins nodded and grinned nervously. He had something else to tell the general. 'I'm afraid that supplies have refused to send up the ammo you sent for, sir. They say it's outdated, expensive and ineffective; usual sort of thing, you know, sir.' He shrugged his shoulders. 'They have sent a list of approved products, if you'd like to see it?'

Practiss grunted and took the paper: another bit of damned bureaucracy. 'What the deuce is this: "Lights, Very, Simple, Green, Officers for the use of." Aren't we allowed any of the multi-coloured sparklers any more? They were the only ones that ever did anything.' He read on, twirling his moustache vigorously. 'And what have we here? They've refused the trench mortars!! Damn it all, they were ideal for bombarding the evacuation trenches. This is absolutely ridiculous. They'll soon be telling us when to change our underpants.'

They set off down the trenches for the morning inspection at breakneck speed, Practiss mumbling under his breath all the way. Only yesterday they'd got a pasting in the next sector from the enemy's heavy litigation brigade, and two weeks ago, they themselves had come under bomb attack from the FPC commando. Damned unpleasant it had been; and now this!

After an hour and a half, they got back to the dugout for a cup of lukewarm cocoa with the rest of the platoon. Perkins looked a bit shocked from the heavy fire that had spattered the trench all morning, and was comforted by the HV, who had a kind heart. The DN had spent the whole morning on tedious paperwork and looked fed up, as he had had no time to see his men yet.

After a short while, Practiss said: 'I would like to discuss the big push. We'll be going over the top at 7 a.m. tomorrow, objective Maladie Grave.' 'Maladie Grave?' Perkins spluttered, his drink spreading across his new uniform in a bright stain. 'I didn't realise that was our objective. I thought this campaign involved preventive fire only.' There was an embarrassed silence in the dugout, only broken by the crump of the guns of the 2nd Opinion Brigade, giving covering fire.

'Actually, Perkins,' Practiss replied, 'we don't always follow the C-in-C's commands to the letter, you know. There's nothing like a little sortie to keep up the men's morale.' 'But sir, isn't Maladie Grave defended by the notorious Trivial Complaints division?' Perkins exclaimed. 'Yes, Perkins, but we can cut through that lot alright,' Practiss replied, smiling at the rest of the team.

Next morning, Practiss stealthily led his men through the wire, over no-man's-land up to the enemy lines. Not a shot was fired. They could even hear the Germans happily talking over their breakfast of Schweinwurstlburgers mit Schlagsahne (pork sausages with whipped cream, delicious, but high in saturated fats). 'OK, Jones. Let 'em have it!' Practiss whispered. Whoosh! A rocket shot up and burst in a cascade of sparks. Out of this floated a red balloon, bucking and swerving in the dank air; and on the balloon, glowing in bright paint, were the words: 'Guter Mann und Gute Frau Clinik.'

'Gott im Himmel!' from the German trench. 'Now go!' Practiss shouted. With the enemy's attention totally diverted by this novelty, the team stormed through the trenches, capturing Maladie Grave with only the lightest of casualties. Practiss was, naturally, very pleased. He had no idea what the German inscription meant: some bright spark in the platoon had read the words in a captured German magazine. The surprise had certainly worked.

The second-in-command, Major Urquhart, arrived back at the front line a week later. He had been on a refresher course back at base and was full of bright ideas. 'We've got to institute performance review, General. It's the only thing they'll talk about at Staff college.' 'And what the deuce is that, Urquhart?' 'Comparison with the neighbouring sectors, General: rate of casualties, use of ammunition, cleanliness of latrines, state of repair of the trenches and so on. It's an exercise in self-flagellation, really: very British. Div. HQ tells me that we don't compare very favourably with the sector on our left.' 'Damn it, Urquhart, they've just got one of the new liaison officers – sector manager, or some such name – damned staff-wallah with good organisational ability. He spends all his time behind a desk, clipping papers. We haven't got one yet.' 'But we have captured Maladie Grave, Major,' Perkins chimed in, cheekily. 'Quite so, Perkins, quite so,' Urquhart replied, trying not to sound too impressed. Individual acts of bravery were not encouraged at Staff College.

Practiss told Urquhart that he would discuss the wretched performance review later, and stomped off to the field telephone post. He was not in a good mood. Erratic supporting fire from their own DHSS guns had resulted in some near misses on their own lines, and the poor DN had been wounded by just one such misdirected barrage yesterday. The MO now informed him that the DN would need transferring to hospital. Lo and behold, when the MO had tried to get him a bed, all the hospitals said they were full!

Now they had managed to get a call through to some hospital miles away. 'Hello!' Practiss shouted. 'Who are you?' The line was very bad. 'Carter-Fortescue. Captain i.c. admin 3rd BMH,' came crackling from the ear-piece. 'Practiss here, General Practiss. Now you listen to me, Cartesqueak. I want our DN admitted immediately; he's got shrapnel wounds in both legs, and is in severe pain.' 'Quite so, General. I understand the situation, but we've got no beds.' 'No beds! Why the devil not?' 'Efficiency drive, General. There are too many casualties at the front. You've really got to be more careful up there.' The line went very crackly. Practiss wasn't sure whether he could have heard the last sentence right.

'Now look here, Cocksqueak. This isn't just anybody you're talking to here, you know: I captured Maladie Grave a week ago. I want this man admitted here and now. The bed shortage is your lookout; my lookout is my men, and I'm ordering you to get him in.' 'Just not possible, General, I'm afraid.' Practiss looked up to the heavens in supplication, then, suddenly, he cupped his hands over the mouthpiece, and whistled stage wind noises down the phone. 'Sorry! Line's very bad, I'll have to ring off,' he gasped, between puffs of the howling gale.

After ten minutes, the phone rang again. It was Corporal Fudgit, from Admissions Division. He was pleased to report that a bed had been found. The DN was to be sent down to the railhead, where a special compartment would be found on the next train down.

'Well done, Corporal,' Practiss shouted, and slammed the phone down again so hard that the handle cracked. 'Marvellous, isn't it? It takes half an hour of negotiation before you can get a wounded man into hospital. Marvellous,' he mumbled to himself. 'Marvellous, sah!' the telephonist dutifully agreed and saluted vigorously.

Perkins, being the most junior officer in the regiment, had been allocated night duty. This meant sitting in the trench all night, watching for any enemy activity and trying to appear authoritative when half asleep. It was boring, tiring, and occasionally frightening work, which was supposed to give the subalterns 'good experience'. Urquhart now did very little of this, making the excuse that he was too busy organising the improved performance during the day to be bothered with getting up at night.

'What about the preventive fire campaign?' Practiss asked Urquhart one morning. 'Are we really achieving any greater success?' 'Actually, General, we've stepped up our rate of fire considerably, and I believe we must be inflicting more casualties. Isn't that right, Perkins?' He nudged Perkins, who had fallen asleep in his chair with a full mug of cocoa on his chest. He had had a hard night on duty. 'Oh, quite so, Major. It is much brighter today,' Perkins mumbled. Practiss nodded. What a thing it was to have keen young officers! He would leave the new-fangled concepts to them, and concentrate on what pleased him most. 'Now listen to this, you two,' he said. 'I've got something very exciting to report. This morning through the binoculars I could just see the Peutz-Jeghers line.' He paused to let the words sink in. 'I intend to take it, come what may,' he said, the stubble bristling on his jutting chin.

Perkins had fallen asleep again, and was beginning to snore loudly. Urquhart nudged him again: the boy had no right to be sleepy. After all, they'd all had to do similar duties in the past, and they'd never fallen asleep on duty. 'We're scheduled for a visit from the C-in-C in two weeks' time,' Practiss continued. 'I'd like to show him what we're capable of.' 'Damned good show,' Urquhart said unenthusiastically. 'But are you quite sure it's the Peutz-Jeghers line?' 'Of course I'm sure. You recognise it by the brown camouflage spots around the gun turrets.' 'Isn't it rather heavily fortified, General?' 'Yes, Urquhart, but I've thought of all that. Now here's the plan . . .' Perkins slumbered on.

Life continued at its normal humdrum pace: long hours of mindless routine, interspersed with occasional jolting excitement as the enemy launched a night raid, or pounded the lines with an artillery barrage. In the middle of one such epidemic of shelling, the DN arrived back, on an early discharge from hospital. He stumbled into the dugout, accompanied by a cloud of dust and cordite.

'Are you fit for duties?' Practiss asked impatiently. He was not an insensitive man, but he had other things on his mind at the present. 'I'm not sure, General. No-one said anything at the hospital.' 'Have you got a letter?' 'Oh no, sir. It's supposed to be coming up later.' 'That's no good: it'll take weeks,' Practiss expostulated. 'I'm sorry, sir, but its apparently part of their efficiency drive,' the DN explained. 'It's more economical to convalesce in the trenches, they said.' 'And what are we supposed to do with you?' 'Oh, I'll manage the best I can,' the DN said cheerily, patting his bad leg, which was still plastered up to the hip.

Practiss took no more notice and returned to his work. He had got together a platoon of ex-miners, who were now tunnelling out from the trench, under no-man's-land, towards the German line. Progress was rather slow, as the ground was wet and heavy clay, rather unsuitable for excavations. Of course news of the enterprise had leaked back to HQ, and was greeted there rather sceptically: another of Practiss's dangerous eccentricities. They sent a telegram from the front:

'Project much too complex. Refer details to base. Will consider appropriate equipment and men.' 'B**** r that. We'll do it our own way,' Practiss exclaimed to his officers, but sent a message back as follows: 'Admirable advice. Details to follow.' The miners redoubled their efforts, and after several days, were under the enemy fortification. Plans were laid for the assault.

Two hours before zero hour; Practiss briefed his team: 'You can expect a spirited defence: the line is occupied by the Polyposis division. They have a reputation of being deadly fighters.' Grim faces in the candlelight of the dugout. 'We have a novel plan, however; it will undoubtedly take them totally by surprise.' 'And us, no doubt,' Urquhart mumbled, *sotto voce.* 'First we hit them with gas,' Practiss continued, 'then, when they are incapacitated, we roll out the hose-pipes.' 'Roll out the hosepipes,' Urquhart repeated to himself, shaking his head. He still had difficulty in believing that this wasn't all a bad dream. 'Their fortifications are totally enclosed, ideal terrain for this sort of thing.' Outside, it was a clear, moonlit night, and shooting stars cut the sky like scissors. An eerie quiet had descended on the battlefield.

At 10.30 p.m., precisely, the guns opened up with a devastating bombardment. The local DHSS commander had refused to get involved, ('against HQ's orders'), but, fortunately, the local BUPA battalion had agreed to support the venture, and its guns were now blasting away with good effect. The shelling lasted a quarter of an hour; meanwhile men and equipment were pouring into the tunnel. At 10.50 p.m., the bombardment changed to gas. Practiss's men were right under the fortifications. With great panache, they now dug upwards, and after ten minutes emerged unscathed inside the German trench system, precisely as the gas shells were taking effect!

The rest is history. Thousands of gallons of water were pumped through pipes laid in the tunnel, so that the sealed dugouts and gun emplacements rapidly flooded. Thus the Germans were flushed out on a tide of water, like flecks of rice in a cholera stool. Outside, they were swiftly captured, sodden and defenceless. Only a few pockets of resistance remained in the line, mostly in the trenches near the surface, and these were dealt with by special teams of Practiss's men, bombing their way along the system.

In two hours, all was in British hands and secured to resist any counter-attack. Practiss sat in a captured bunker, drinking Schnapps and feeling proud of himself. He said to the field telephonist: 'Send this telegram to HQ, Wheeler: "Request visit to the front now to discuss further details re Peutz-Jeghers plan. Surprising development re your estimation 'over-ambitious'. Practiss, i.c. Polyposis div."'

The C-in-C's visit to the front took place ten days later. Field

Marshall Moore-Orless ('More for Less' to all the army), was a suave man, with boyish, handsome features, who was supposed to be great favourite with the King himself. His rise through the ranks had been meteoric, leaving a stream of jealousies and resentments in his wake, and, although somewhat dogged by ill-health, he had assembled an enthusiastic team under him, who were promoting his policy with relish, as long as they were certain what that policy was. Accompanying him today was the elegant figure of Brigadier Edward Favour, Chief of Staff, who was even younger and more handsome, and always in the best of health, and who never lost an opportunity to express his point of view in the most forthright of terms.

Even General Practiss was a little nervous, and Major Urquhart was positively quaking in his boots. Second Lieutenant Perkins, however, in his youthful naïvety, was looking forward to meeting them all. Urquhart had made sure that the latrines gleamed and smelt of distant pinewoods, and the trench sandbags were faultlessly aligned. He had also prepared reams of figures on preventive fire, and was ready to talk for twenty minutes on the subject, if called upon, which everyone prayed he wouldn't be.

As it turned out, however, the visit was somewhat of an anti-climax. Moore-Orless seemed preoccupied, and Favour spent his time inspecting the field kitchens (which Urquhart had forgotten to tidy up), making derogatory comments about the standard of food in the trenches. The capture of the Peutz-Jeghers line seemed only of passing interest: Moore-Orless was impressed that Practiss had managed the whole attack on his own initiative – 'damned plucky' he called it – but was more interested that the BUPA battalion had agreed to give covering fire. He made no apologies for the lack of support from the DHSS battalion. The last thing that Perkins saw was the BUPA commander talking animatedly with the C-in-C.

That's gratitude,' Perkins said, when they had all gone. 'We might as well have not made the effort,' Urquhart agreed. The DN looked seriously depressed. His leg was still hurting a lot.

General Practiss thrust his hands deep into his pockets and shrugged. 'Ah well,' he said, 'we don't do it all for the C-in-C, do we?' At that, he pulled a pipe out from his pocket, and strode off to inspect his men.

After he'd gone, Perkins said: 'He's got guts, hasn't he, Major?' 'Hmmm,' murmured Urquhart. He was very disappointed that no-one had bothered to look at his preventive figures. Perkins shrugged his shoulders and climbed out of the dugout. He knew where his loyalties lay.

NICHOLAS DUNN
Poole

Progress

(Tune from *HMS Pinafore*)

When I was a lad I served a term
  As junior houseman on a GI firm,
I wrote the records and I worked till late
And I treated indigestion with trisilicate,
I treated indigestion so successfully
That now I am a highly qualified GP

As house physician I earned such esteem
That I gained admission to a training scheme,
In Casualty I took great pride
In giving the dyspeptics metaclopramide.
Their heartfelt thanks encouraged me
To hope to be a highly qualified GP

That A and E job soon came to an end
On obstetrics next I had six months to spend
When the ladies of heartburn did complain
I found that alginate relieved their pain.
Then I sat for the DRCOG
So I could be a highly qualified GP

I left obstetrics when I'd made my name
And a geriatrician I then became.
Hiatus hernia patients ceased to moan
Their reflux cured with carbenoxolone.
Such quick relief I could guarantee
That I'd soon become a highly qualified GP

And after this to my lot it befell
In surgery to spend my final spell.
I cut down all the operating lists
By healing ulcers with H_2 antagonists.
The senior surgeon recommended me
To hurry up and qualify as a GP

My scheme completed, all that now remained
Was a year in practice to be fully trained.
I found it was my trainer's will
To treat bad stomachs with mist. mag. trisil.
When I learned that most were soon pain-free
I knew I had begun to be a real GP

MARIE CAMPKIN
London

2
Doctors Talking with Patients

People are more aware of their guts than any other organ in the body; not surprisingly, as upsets in function are liable to occur unexpectedly at any time and age. Traveller's diarrhoea, heartburn and constipation are, for example, no respecters of persons. Furthermore, the owner can influence his or her guts by the food that is eaten or tablets swallowed. Hence patients tend to make their own diagnoses which may mislead: 'heartburn' often has nothing to do with the correct definition, 'biliousness' is unrelated to the liver or biliary system and 'wind' covers various sensations from belching to feelings of fullness. 'What do you complain of?' the doctor might ask. 'Gastric stomach', replies the patient.

The problem of communication lies at the heart of medicine: for diagnosis and successful doctor–patient relationships depend upon the art of listening and speaking to patients. But the language is different and the vernacular is needed to help understanding; misunderstandings and malapropisms often arise.

The Things They Say   (I)

The student was taking his first history and was extremely embarrassed at the intimacy of the questions he was supposed to ask. How did one put questions about bowel function to elderly ladies one had never met before?

Taking a deep breath he plunged in with 'are your bowels open regularly?'

She was far less perturbed than he: 'Oh, yes quite regular; every Saturday morning.'

'Good Lord! Do you take anything?'

'Oh yes, I always take my knitting.'

ROBIN HULL
Birmingham

The Things They Say (II)

The little old Cockney lady exposed her abdomen for examination. It was a veritable battlefield, criss-crossed with the scars of many a surgical encounter over her eighty years. Seeing the young doctor's astonishment she gave him a conducted tour.

Her nicotined fingers indicated the right hypochondrium: 'this was for gall' she explained, and 'this was where they did me ulster'. Her hand moved lower, first in the midline, then in the right iliac fossa as she added 'this was where it were all took away, and this was the first one, the benedict.'

Then she coyly drew down the calico of her nether underwear revealing the grey wisps adorning her ancient mons veneris and, leering salaciously added 'and this, ah this, was me hopperation for rapture.'

ROBIN HULL
Birmingham

If Richard Brinsley Sheridan had, in his play 'The Rivals', portrayed Mrs Malaprop as being costive, she might have said she was taking laxatives for her vowels, or using rectal apostles or prudential enemas.

Getting to the Bottom of it All

The general practitioner's association with the bowels begins with the digestion of large amounts of information at medical school. Quite often this intellectual nutrition is in a high fibre form; much of it is unabsorbed and goes straight through.

At university one learns all those medical terms that allow one to converse with other doctors. Unfortunately, less emphasis is placed upon communicating with the people to whom those medical labels become attached, that is, the patients. So the impersonal 'There's an interesting spleen in bed six' is used instead of saying 'Mr Bloggs the window cleaner.' Generations of students have toyed with their new vocabularies to produce humour that becomes engrained in the medical school furniture: for example, there is a professorial chair in cardiology but only a stool of gastroenterology.

Often, undergraduate textbooks tell the story of a particular case and the students must deduce the diagnosis from the information given. The only one of these that I can recall was the case where the patient had a 'blockage' and a hard mass was felt in the abdomen. Surely, a look into the bowel from below would confirm the suspicion that this poor patient had a tumour? Not so. In the secular science of medicine nothing is obvious. Turning the formalin-stained pages of the anatomy book revealed a surprise solution to the problem. In cold clinical terms the text declared, 'at operation a small vase, bearing the inscription "a present from Rockport" was found.' Our student group immediately resolved never to holiday in Rockport.

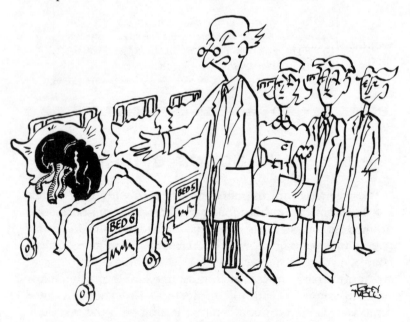

There's an interesting spleen in bed six

The intestine is more than a hollow inner tube. It is a complex organ of many different parts that must be peered at through the microscope. It was a bit disappointing to discover that the 'Crypts of Lieberkühn' are just another part of the bowel, rather than the haunt of a certain Transylvanian count. With time, the future GP moves from the lecture room to the hospital. Here you meet the living and learn how to keep them that way. With the expansion of medical schools, clinical material, also known as patients, has become scarce in some areas. I was yawning away in a consultant's clinic when the surgeon discovered that neither of the somnolent students in his clinic had performed a rectal examination while attached to his ward. He immediately ordered the patient to remove his trousers so that we could perform this invasive procedure for the first time. The patient probably never came back for his toenail operation.

As a clinical student I was asked to escort a patient to the X-ray Department for a picture to be taken to find the cause of her tummy pain. The film showed a veritable scrap-yard of swallowed metal. How can a pair of knitting needles be swallowed when a stomach is already full of pins, tacks and screws? No wonder she had pains. I am sure that if we had laid this patient on the floor she would have pointed North.

Children are more prone to swallowing objects accidentally. Most medical staff can give accounts of the articles they have retrieved. There is the story of the little boy who swallowed a half-crown. When an anxious relative telephoned the hospital enquiring about the patient the reply was 'There has been no change yet.' With inflation, I suppose this anecdote probably now involves a £1 coin.

The way that various items get lost in those twenty-seven feet of intestine is amazing. The patient often knows the nature of the problem but is too embarrassed to tell the doctor: one patient with pain in the lower part of the belly was admitted to hospital. When a stethoscope was placed on the abdomen a strange humming noise was heard emanating from within. This caused intense diagnostic debate, as the patient was giving no clues. The mystery was not solved until an operation discovered a lost vibrator.

Leaving the red-brick walls of the hospital behind, one soon learns that medical matters are not so clear-cut in general practice.

Patients complain of 'gastric stomach' or 'cardiac heart'. Like a Klondyke prospector the GP must sift through a lot of material to find the nugget.

Patients give graphic descriptions of their tummy pains; 'like a hot poker'; 'like a rat gnawing inside'. One wonders how many of these patients have endured the experience to which they are comparing their pain? Just the other day a patient complained that she felt as though she was being 'digested by enzymes'. This description was clearly based on an advertisement for a biological washing powder which showed little green enzymes munching their way through the weekly wash. Those PR men have a lot to answer for.

These days, everyone can experience travel to foreign parts. Often tropical diseases are brought home and perplex the local GP. Diarrhoea is a common duty-free import. The GP must find out if Spanish Tummy is different to Montezuma's Revenge. Is the cause of Delhi Belly the same bug as Bali Belly? Are the runs more severe than the trots? But you do not have to leave these shores to be food-poisoned, as some hospital authorities know very well. I once dealt with an outbreak of Salmonella in a plush hotel. After a sumptuous dinner, every hour saw a guest succumb to the bug and another call to my surgery. I hope that the manager did not think I was being ungrateful when I declined the offer of a free meal as a reward for my work.

Toddlers can cause havoc out of all proportion to their size. They soon learn that their bowels are a formidable weapon. Adults may think that toilet training is about teaching the toddler; however, it can be the toddler who calls the tune. Smart toddlers quickly realise that by choosing the right time and place to deposit their load, they soon have their parents proferring promises and rewards. When you do not get your own way, why waste all that energy throwing a temper tantrum, when filling your nappy is such an effective protest that it can't be ignored. *This* is potty power. Children who go through this stage of despotism, perhaps we should say

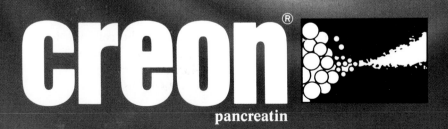

despottysm, probably become captains of industry or politicians, on account of their manipulative skills.

The guts of general practice often involves trying to alter the lifestyles of the patients in order to benefit their health, which is much harder than prescribing a pill. Encouragement of weight loss is a familiar task. Many grossly obese patients respond to my maxim 'you are what you eat', with the reply 'I don't eat a thing, Doctor.' This is obviously untrue, but I am usually put in my place with 'I think it's my glands Doctor': glands that are so powerful that they cause people who eat 'nothing' to break the surgery scales.

The digestive system can present the GP with a large part of the practice workload. Due to experience ranging from bilious babies to grannies with gripe your doctor can be relied upon to get to the *bottom* of the matter.

J. DOWDEN
Rotorua, New Zealand

Borborygmus

Borborygmi. Borborygmi. Onomatopoeia is the gut reaction that says it all. Take 'Mum' in any language and you can hear that chomp as the blessed little mite finds the nipple. Glug and gulp hardly count as proper words, but borborygmi—further down the scale, so to speak—there's a name to conjure with. The Greeks had a word for almost everything and lots of them have descended into modern English without the average native here having a clue where they came from. They would have died out long ago if it wasn't for onomatopoeia instilled in us from birth and perhaps even before birth. What a glorious idea: subliminal advertising by bowel sounds to the unborn twins from an expectant world around them. Heart beats and borborygmi to soften the battering they might otherwise hear from civilisation. Sufficient peace and then reassuringly tonic messages tom-tomming in the tum-tum of Mum. A lullaby of lovely loose logic. Facts of fart. *Cogito, ergo tum* is the melodic motto of motions masticated methodically with the mood.

More's the pity, then, that so much of what we say in surgery is too quickly dismissed by patients as jargon. 'Could you just tell me', said a spritely great mound of flesh to my rather athletic secretary after I had been explaining to her in words of one syllable why the flab was there, 'what's a Mentum?' As this was not immediately clear, my secretary said she would find out and let the patient know. I had no recollection of using a two-syllable word at all, let alone one as long as omentum–or as mystifying to the uninitiated. I had so carefully avoided reference to the Krebs Cycle. (I had once tried to explain it to a diabetic BA(Hons) patient but forgot the famous story of the Oxford don who was found pumping up his bicycle by the wrong tyre's valve – upon being challenged by a group of passing fellows, he replied, 'What? Do they not communicate?') This otherwise intuitive and sensitive patient of mine had thought that I was trying to get him to eat more sugar so that he should be fit enough for the Tour de France. Metabolic pathways are roads to hell paved with good intentions when it comes to one-to-one biology tutorials rather than good old-fashioned keep-taking-the-tablets didacticism. 'The apron of the stomach' instead of omentum, and 'your flabby bits' are phrases that spring to mind perhaps using two syllables apiece but they had never been linked in the mind that mattered. O, Men-tum, what did she think you were? Did she think I meant she was about to change sex? She never came back.

I had an antipodean encounter in my house job days with a Maori who thought the lines on her abdomen were so-called because they were 'stray'. Umbilicus has always resounded in my mind as a word that should have originated in Pidgin: as the pot is being brought to the boil the sigh of resignation goes up from the unfortunate future fare, about to be turned into long pig, and he mutters, 'M'Bi like us.' And so, full circle back to the womb. Boom! goes onomatopoeia again. Dark, cosy and unfathomably mysterious, it resonates with more to come. 'Bottom' is such an anticlimax. 'Down below' is ambivalent, depending on the way it is said. 'Bowels' are nearly there, but nothing can beat borborygmi for me. They are so unutterably plural. Give me low-sounding jargon any day.

MICHAEL JAMESON
St Albans

The Motto

There are many homes whose living room proudly displays a board bearing words of significance and thought. Often it is framed and competes on the walls with copies of Landseer's 'Monarch of the Glen' or Constable's 'Hay Wain'. The motto varies from the religious ('God is Love') to the sentimental ('Home Sweet Home'). To a casual caller such messages can be quite helpful – little clues to the personality of the householder and, perhaps, allowing suitable openings for decorous conversation.

This situation was rather specialised in the house of my nice old patient Fred. He, unfortunately, suffered from Diverse Ticklosis, which is what he believed it was called. My partners and I thought of it more correctly as Diverticulosis. In his case it was not severe, causing only occasional, but annoying, bowel looseness.

Fred's attacks responded quickly, nicely, to a good old routine pharmaceutical preparation. When bothered he would make an appointment to get a new prescription for the stuff, we would have a little chat and off he would go. Eventually he stopped calling and just sent a polite note requesting a new supply of his 'diarrhoea medicine'. We both missed the gossip but we saved a lot of time and he knew that if recovery was not fast he should, and would, come to see me at once.

The snag was that Fred was no orthographist, especially concerning a word like 'diarrhoea'. It is a difficult term to spell and no one can be blamed for getting it wrong. Our practice got quite used to receiving a note asking for 'Diurea', 'Dyorra', 'Direa' or 'Direrear' medicines. We understood what he meant.

Now Fred realised perfectly well that he never quite got it right and this bothered him. And then, at last, he told me that he had had the word elegantly copied from a dictionary onto a notice and so, in the future, would manage correctly.

He did not; crazy spellings still came in with his requests. Fred apologised and said that the copied word never seemed to be in the right place when he needed to consult it.

One day (when I was visiting his wife) I saw the famous notice. Very prominent on the centre of the living room mantelpiece stood a large decorative card carrying in bold capitals the message 'DIARRHOEA'. I wondered just how much this dominating feature among the other knick-knacks could affect social events in his home. I congratulated Fred on the accuracy and emphasis of the notice. But I suggested how much more appropriate it might be to move it to another and altogether different room.

A.S. PLAYFAIR
Cambridge

'More mistakes are made from want of a proper examination than for any other reason' goes the aphorism. But perhaps a statistical investigation might show that lack of a proper history comes first. Doctors who deal with patients having trouble with their guts often have a problem: the victim has to be undressed.

First, Find Your Patient

I reckon that general practice has never been the same since the advent of the slim-fit shirt. There was a time when the male physique could become totally available within seconds. Off with the jacket, slip down the braces, lift up the shirt and then, with a flick of the top trouser button, Homo Sapiens (male) was revealed in all his glory. Fat or thin, it made no difference. Now, alas, the shirt is contoured to the shape and retained in place by at least twenty-three small buttons closely opposed to the chest and a further two at each cuff. Many an appointment system has foundered on the impenetrable slim-fit shirt.

As if that wasn't bad enough, other tightly occlusive garments followed. Jeans are truly anatomical – even if their physiology leaves something to be desired. As a result, abdominal examination has become a difficult, time-consuming and, occasionally, dangerous art. To make matters worse, increasing numbers of patients are wearing clothes the upper and lower parts of which are welded together or 'all in one'. Even babies are no longer easily available to the examining hand by the simple means of dividing their clothes in the middle. Now there is an outer layer that occludes them from finger tip to toe. Underneath that is a one-piece 'jogging suit' and finally there is the dreaded vest–pant combination.

For a while, the impact of these garments on the GP's time/ efficiency ratio was reduced by the passing fashion in young women of being harry starkers under their jogging suits. This not only allowed you to make up some lost time, but avoided the risks to the hands of unwary physicians occasioned by the sudden rolling of a panty girdle.

But then came that most obscenely inelegant foundation garment, the all-in-one crutch-fastening corset. The first time I came face to face with one I knew that a disaster was inevitable and it was no surprise that that disaster, when it came, came to big Grace Wilson. 'Amazing Grace' is a walking miracle. Not only has she borne her life-long mysterious and excruciating abdominal pain with fortitude, she has borne it without any obvious ill effect on her health. She can get to doctors that other patients cannot reach. In fog and snow and ice and hurricane, she will keep her appointment when others fail.

But her appearance that afternoon was unusual. There was something restrained about her entry. Her face was a trifle suffused and she sat down slowly and carefully. I thought I could detect, with my naked ear, a pleural creak as she breathed. Her usual outpourings were more stilted than ever before and she occasionally paused for breath. I decided that it was time for another thorough examination and asked her to retire behind the screen to prepare herself. There was much grunting and panting and scrabbling of clothes. Time passed. Her efforts increased and I began to fear for her health. Suddenly–pop-pop-pop. Then a great rush of noise like the rolling up of a Venetian blind and finally a choking, strangled cry. I rushed behind the screen to find her already in the terminal stages of strangulation. Her all-in-one, its fierce tension released, had catapulted up her mighty torso, thrown her arms above her head and now encircled her neck. With aplomb, I divided the encircling garment with a handy scalpel. She relaxed, straightened her hair, climbed up on the couch and said 'It's

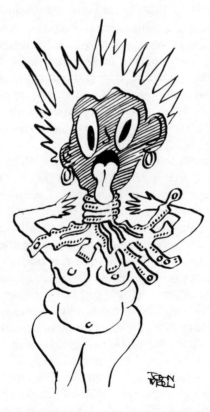

Her all-in-one had catapulted up her mighty torso, thrown her arms above her head and now encircled her neck.

here, doctor', indicating her left side. 'It's no better.' The consultation continued along the usual lines.

Amazing woman, our Grace.

RONALD MULROY
Wakefield

The Patient's Song
(Tune: *The London Derrière*)

Oh Doctor Roy, my pipes, my pipes are stalling,
  I think I've got a blockage here inside.
I should have gone–the pain is quite appalling
  But still the call to stool's unsatisfied.
So I've come back to plead for your attention,
  My haemorrhoids are all prolapsed below,
I've taken pills, more times than I can mention,
  Oh Doctor Roy, Oh Doctor Roy, I need you so.

But if you turn a deaf ear to my crying,
  When I am dead, as dead I well may be,
Don't think that you'll escape your fate by lying
  When you're reported to the GMC.
So just think twice before you try rejecting me,
  Don't you neglect my sigmoidoscopy,
With legal aid the lawyers are protecting me
  And you will get no peace till you take care of me.

MARIE CAMPKIN
London

3
Odd Tastes and Objects Swallowed

D r Frank Buckland, who qualified at St George's Hospital in 1851 but forsook medicine to write and continue zoological research, was a gourmet with unusual tastes in food. Crocodile was sometimes served to guests or mice cooked in butter, the nastiest thing that he ate being a mole and the next worst a bluebottle.[1]

Tastes more odd than these may arise during normal pregnancy: some may yearn for watercress while others enjoy munching coal – preferring the black shiny type as it tastes more crisp and nutty. Other patients may swallow objects either accidentally (see later, The Troubles of Rotarian Church) or deliberately. For example:

A middle-aged women with nervous symptoms complained that she had difficulty in swallowing. Her doctor diagnosed globus hystericus and told her that it was 'the change', as she was at the menopause; but antidepressants had no effect and she got worse. Oesophagoscopy showed that the GP was – in a way – correct: because several coins, the change that she had received when shopping, were retrieved.

The record achieved by a compulsive swallower was awarded by the Guiness Book of Records (1988) to an insane woman of forty-two years who complained of 'slight abdominal pain'. She had swallowed two thousand, five hundred and thirty-three objects including nine hundred and forty-seven bent pins – all of which lay in her stomach.

Medico-legal problems may arise. The doctor who looked after Henry King was fortunate (as the writer suggests) in not being sued for medical negligence. The boy's case history was as follows:

Henry King

Who chewed bits of String, and was early cut off in Dreadful Agonies.

The Chief Defect of Henry King
Was chewing little bits of String.
At last he swallowed some which tied
Itself in ugly Knots inside.

Physicians of the Utmost Fame
Were called at once; but when they came
They answered, as they took their Fees,
'There is no Cure for this Disease.
Henry will very soon be dead.'
His Parents stood about his Bed
Lamenting his Untimely Death,
When Henry, with his Latest Breath,
Cried—'Oh, my Friends, be warned by me,
That Breakfast, Dinner, Lunch and Tea
Are all the Human Frame requires...'
With that, the Wretched Child expires.

HILAIRE BELLOC
In *Cautionary Tales*

The Kordelbezoar of Henry King

There can be few more startling cases of medical negligence than the unfortunate plight of Henry King, so movingly described by Hilaire Belloc. The child should not, of course, have been allowed to persist with his dangerous habit of chewing string – granted too that his parents, before the days of the NHS general practitioner, were forced to go to the private sector for advice – yet despite these deficiencies the young patient deserved better treatment.

Why did Henry die? It is reported that the string he swallowed 'tied itself in ugly knots inside', but there is no postmortem evidence that obstruction from this *kordelbezoar* led to his demise. In fact, the end was remarkably swift, following immediately after the delivery of a clearly stated homily on the dangers of his fatal habit. One can only assume that the intra-abdominal ball of string was so huge that it led to pressure on his inferior vena cava producing a deep vein thrombosis from which he suffered a catastrophic and theatrically timed pulmonary embolism.

It is debatable whether Master King's life was salvageable in his final throes. There is, however, clear evidence that his medical advisers – the number of whom involved is uncertain from Mr Belloc's account – were guilty of the most appalling errors of management during the early stages of his illness. It says very little for the quality of the profession in his lifetime, for we are told that 'physicians of the *utmost fame* were called at once' (my italics). Here I think the story is inaccurate. Mr and Mrs King would surely not have summoned these eminent doctors all together, but would in desperation have sought second, third and fourth opinions, as the prognosis offered each time was so gloomy. Were the physicians in collusion? Did each recommend the next as he departed? We shall never know. They did, however, make two statements at the end of their visits, one accurate but the other totally wrong. That Henry would die soon was exactly what happened. That there was no cure for his disease was quite untrue because he could and should have had a laparotomy.

Now we come to the question of fees and here there is clear evidence that the physicians were working together. A surgeon would speedily have removed the obstruction and brought the case to a satisfactory close. But milking the Kings with a stream of successive *medical* opinions ensured the syndicate of a much greater income. Henry ought to have had an autopsy, but the bereaved parents were obviously too distraught to ask for one. The doctors got off scot free and wealthier. The Kings lost a considerable proportion of their family fortune in addition to their string-chewing, but otherwise innocent, son.

An enquiry into this scandalous case of malpractice is long overdue. It should be carried out by Miss Esther Rantzen and the *That's Life* team, who after their mauling at the hands of Dr Sidney Gee will be out for revenge.

JOHN WOODWARD
Sidcup

And a case of 'Pot Belly' illustrates a new purpose in swallowing objects.

A thirty-three-year-old man attended the Accident and Emergency Department saying that he had swallowed eighteen condoms filled with hashish to get the drug through the customs. He had attended A and E departments in two other hospitals but stated that nothing had been done since his story was not believed. Since then, he had recovered only twelve, two being vomited and ten having passed rectally which is the usual way for these smugglers to recover their booty. X-rays showed six filling defects and a deformed duodenal cap, suggesting that the foreign bodies were unlikely to go further; he had previously suffered from a duodenal ulcer. To forestall possible disintegration of the contraceptive sheaths and a potentially lethal overdose of hashish, the surgeon, with the patient's written consent, operated and not only removed the six packets but also performed a vagotomy and pyloroplasty.

The police brought charges against the patient, who had given written permission for the surgeon to disclose his medical history to them. The police expressed surprise that the surgeon had not reported the facts to them, but as there was no threat to 'life or limb' of others, the doctor had no duty to break confidentiality with the patient.[2]

4
Persistent Belly Ache: a Nightmare for Patients and for Doctors

Its this damned belly that gives a man his worst troubles

HOMER
c. 850 BC[3]

A bdominal pain – where belly ache persists although a complete examination and relevant investigations fail to show any cause – is a bane for doctors, and, of course, for patients. The irritable bowel, called furious bowel by the woman in the following case history, explains many cases and this abnormal motility (or spasm) may affect any part of the alimentary tract, even the gullet and stomach.

A Gut Feeling

I plough placidly through the viral or emotional sniffles of evening surgery on Automatic Doctor, until I notice that Mrs P. is my next patient. A sweet, elderly and very fit widow, cheerful despite her numerous complaints, she passes her lonely hours by inventing gastrointestinal syndromes, then presenting them to me in insoluble form. We have played this game for years. In my more naïve days, it worried me that I never seemed to progress with her down any definite medical pathway; all attempts to investigate, categorise or treat were thwarted. On each visit, the loop of her intestine which I felt around my neck tightened, slowly throttling me into helplessness. Then, a few appointments short of asphyxiation, I extinguished the notion of medical intervention, realising that my role was simply that of listener: no more, no less. She complains, I sympathise, we both remain happy. Now I tend to use this ear service as a thin cover to allow myself an indulgent period of consultation-length daydreaming; this I dutifully, but vainly, try to resist, although I hope that my interested expression and concerned grunts, which punctuate her interminable symptom roll-call, might conceal my true cerebral activity.

Ushering her into the surgery, I notice that one hand is already clamped ominously on her abdomen, ready to indicate the site of the latest pain or gurgle. Slowly, she sits down, a mischievous grin on her face: Mrs P. and her performing bowel. She apologises, as ever, for being a nuisance, then launches into her soliloquy.

It's the old tummy trouble doctor . . .

I lean back in my chair, switch on my concerned expression, and hope that body-language and the statutory 'hmms' and 'uh-uhs' will suffice.

I . . . I just can't keep a thing down . . .

The devil on my shoulder, who enjoys these occasions, starts to divert my thoughts.

. . . you should hear the rumbling . . .

What was it last time? Ah yes, gastrointestinal titles, or gastro-intestitles. I recall a few: 'The Diarrhoea of a Provincial Lady', Homer's Ileum, anything by Arthur Colon Doyle or Sigmoid Freud . . .

. . . and as for my tail end, well . . .

I search the recesses of my memory in vain. Other specialities seem more fertile. I switch to the dermatological ('Wart and Peace'), the gynaecological ('Womb with a View') and, finally, the respiratory ('Great Expectorations'), before I mentally travel the entire length of the gut, seeking further inspiration. I arrive, conveniently, at the anus.

. . . and I'm suffering so much flatulence . . .

Of course: 'Fart from the Madding Crowd'. My mask slips into a smile for a moment and Mrs P. pauses. I freeze. She scans my face, which instantly reverts to earnest attentiveness.

Apparently satisfied, she continues, and the devil on my shoulder gives a relieved belly laugh.

. . .but something else is wrong down below now . . .

Belly laugh . . . I ponder on examples of intestinally orientated phrases in common usage. Sick of, it turns my stomach, fed up, gutted, I can't stomach it, bellyacher . . .

. . . and I seem to be passing blood quite often . . .

. . . butterflies in the stomach, gut feeling. Gut feeling. Perhaps I am unusually alert. Possibly I am feeling a shade neglectful of Mrs P. Probably it is last night's curry. Whatever the reason, I receive a gut feeling. It is mixed with guilt and it hurts. I haven't examined Mrs P. for years, not since the days when each consultation fuelled my frustration and ended with mumbled platitudes and a pat on her head or abdomen, depending on my diligence. The devil on my shoulder has been replaced by an angel who reminds me, wearily, that if I don't put my finger in it, I'll put my foot in it. There have been dark times with Mrs P. when I would gladly have introduced my foot to her rectum, or thereabouts, in the hope that the associated discomfort might precipitate her departure and discourage her from returning. As she obligingly adopts the left lateral position, I mutter soothingly and introduce my jellied finger.

What is that? Just for a moment, I receive the Braille impression of a tumour which then scuttles away malignantly to some dark, unreachable rectal corner. I can picture it there, grinning and making obscene gestures at me. I am convinced and wonder what to say to the flummoxed Mrs P., who hurriedly makes herself presentable again, pink with the post-rectal flush.

Gently, I tell her I would like her to see a specialist to sort out the bleeding. In the same breath, I insist that there is nothing to worry about. The devil has returned, and it points out that this is false reassurance, that I am talking nonsense, and that, interestingly, nonsense can issue from either of the two gastro-intestinal apertures: one can talk utter crap, or speak from one's anal orifice. It also tells me that, apart from any significant pathology, Mrs P. undoubtedly has verbal diarrhoea. I ignore all this and swat the devil from my shoulder.

Mrs P. hurries from my surgery, her usually cheerful countenance transformed into frightened confusion. She leaves behind a rather frightened and confused doctor.

For the next few days, I suffer the various well-described stages of a bereavement reaction. My initial shock at the uncovering of pathology is replaced by denial: I didn't feel a tumour. I didn't do a rectal examination. Mrs P. isn't my patient. I am not a doctor. Then I feel angry. How could her rectum do this to me? How could her intestines lull me into a false sense of polysymptomatic security, only to gleefully pull the rug from under my feet? The anger I feel most intensely is directed towards myself for my sin of omission. How long has that growth hidden there, camouflaged by the rest of the bowel's diversionary tactics? An earlier examination might have resulted in earlier diagnosis and an improved prognosis. She always seemed so perfectly fit; she slotted so conveniently into the category of the 'well complainer'. Would others have done differently? Should I have listened more? To cope with these uncomfortable feelings, I enter the bargaining stage. Dear God or Mr Surgeon, whichever is applicable (to many, they are synonymous): please deliver Mrs P. back to me safely, preferably without a colostomy, and I promise to listen to every word she says in future, do a PR on each visit and screen my entire practice population for faecal occult bloods.

For weeks, I hear nothing. Mrs P. is conspicuously absent, each day, from my surgery list. I pretend to enjoy the fact that I have at last escaped from her bowels and I try to concentrate my efforts on other demanding patients. But as time passes and still she does not appear, I become anxious and progressively more guilt-ridden. Has something awful happened? Emergency surgery? Terminal care? Death, even? I start to suffer nightmares: her guts play the ultimate dirty trick on her by feigning illness for so long that she starts to ignore them. Then, without warning, they turn inside out and enzymatically devour her. This dream recurs and I soon become its subject. The enzymes I detect so palpably are the cold sweats which bathe me by the time I wake, panic stricken.

Life becomes miserable: the sight of bottles of laxatives makes me tearful. My family notice that I go very quiet during toilet-roll commercials. The thought of anti-emetics makes me feel sick. The other partners in the practice detect the change in me as I trudge lifelessly around. Finally, I admit that I miss her.

I am visited by a drug representative. He is marketing 'Happigut', a pill which, he claims, will cure all the ills of the gastrointestinal tract, from peptic ulcer to piles. By festooning me with graphs and figures, he tries to convince me of Happigut's

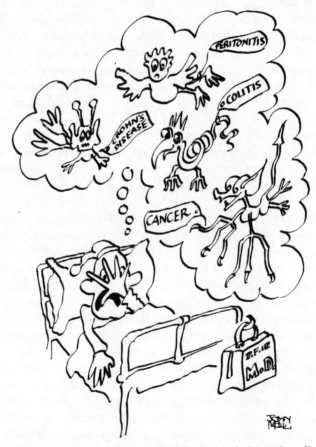

The nightmare of a doctor who is worried that he is missing serious disease in a woman with many neurotic symptoms.

efficacy. I am only half listening, engrossed in my own misery, aware that neither Happigut nor any other wonder drug can do much for poor Mrs P. Eventually I interrupt by asking him if he has anything for depression. He looks confused, thrusts a biro in my direction and bustles away.

The irony of this meeting is not lost on the more impenetrable recesses of my brain. As a result, I suffer another nightmare, even more bizarre, lurid and disturbing than the last.

I am a Happigut tablet. Having been shaken from my container, I am thrust into someone's gaping mouth, mercifully swallowed whole rather than chewed. A sensation of falling, then slowing, then a thud. I sit up and look around. I am in the stomach. Initially, it is too dark to see and I have no torch or matches. Gradually, I perceive a few shapes: they look like lunch remnants, so I guess that it is probably early afternoon. Then I bump into another couple of Happigut tablets. We are the only ones around, so, thankfully, an overdose seems unlikely. Initially nervous, like strangers waiting in an airport departure lounge, we later relax, have a drink and play some pool. I am introduced to a Contraceptive Pill, who tells me that she was swallowed accidentally, due to the stomach owner's combination of severe headache, short-sightedness and pill-taking daughter. Since she is relatively redundant in what, she informs me, is an old lady's infertile body, she has decided to treat the event as a vacation and indulge in some sightseeing. We are discussing plans when a sudden spasm lurches us out of the pylorus and onto a glorious helter-skelter through the duodenum. We laugh, exhilarated, as each peristaltic wave sends us flying along the slippery mucosa, and having bile squirted in our faces does little to dampen our spirits. So much do we enjoy the ride that we consider taking the enterohepatic circulation to repeat the experience.

But things soon turn sour. As we approach the ileum, we meet a tetracycline tablet slouching moodily against a villus. The Contraceptive Pill is quite taken by him, and, recalling the well-documented interactions between contraceptives and tetracyclines, I decide to leave them to it. The ileum is tortuous, dark and slimy. After an age, I reach what I guess is the ileocaecal junction, but here I lose my way; there is nowhere to buy a map and I have no compass. I guess incorrectly, arrive in a cul-de-sac and have to turn back. As luck would have it, a tomato skin passes by, so I hitch a lift. The going gets stodgier as we progress through the colon.

'Here we are, the end of the road,' announces the tomato skin, coming to a halt. We have reached the rectum. Realising that I have arrived intact, totally undigested, I make a mental note never to prescribe Happigut and I resolve to take the drug representative to task on this matter in due course. Cautiously, I grope around, for the darkness is inky and vile. I freeze with horror as I bump into something large and fleshy.

'Watch it' it snarls. 'Leave me alone.'

A piece of sweetcorn sidles reassuringly up to me. 'Don't mind him,' it soothes, 'just a miserable old rectal cancer.' I shiver. The sweetcorn and its companions tell me that they have been waiting around down here for about three days; apparently, yesterday, a plastic tube appeared inexplicably from somewhere outside and sprayed noxious fluid everywhere. As a result, many of them were swept to their doom. Naturally, all this does little for my growing sense of nausea. We sit around like condemned prisoners, swapping stories with artificial joviality, awaiting the final expulsive effort and our awful fate. I remember that I cannot swim.

Longer and longer we wait.

Suddenly: screams. Mayhem. A glinting scalpel blade slices effortlessly through tissue layers just beside me. Light blinds my eyes. I hear the rectal cancer howl. Blood is everywhere. I scramble out through the wound, vault over the surgeons and race out of the operating theatre. In total panic, I hurtle down the corridor; I hear them chasing me and I glance around. All clear. I turn a corner and run straight into a huge policeman. He handcuffs me and drags me into a room in which sit some faceless people. The rest of the room is bare. I am too exhausted to protest and I have difficulty concentrating as they speak but I pick out words which seem to be repeated endlessly: complaint, hearing, negligent, GMC, punishment. Punishment: this is inevitable and awful. My head hangs in shame. I am to be disembowelled.

Next morning. I wake, grateful to escape my sickening dream world. Hurriedly, I open my medical bag and snatch my stethoscope. Flinching as I place the diaphragm on my abdomen, I wait patiently. There it is: a reassuring gurgle. All is well. Then I phone my defence body to check that my subscriptions are up to date.

One month later: evening surgery. To my astonishment, Mrs P.'s name appears halfway down my list. The preceding patients are dealt with in perfunctory manner until I wait, in agony, for Mrs P. to appear.

The return of the mischievous grin. She is sorry to be a nuisance; she has delayed this visit to be sure that I have all the information from the hospital. She sits happily, politely, as I check through her notes. The Consultant's letter, scarcely able to conceal its mirth, tells me that what was, presumably, a piece of 'faecal material' foxed me into believing that Mrs P. had a carcinoma of the rectum. The devil on my shoulder points out that not only did I talk crap, I also felt it. And the bleeding? This was caused, quite simply, by piles, the letter giggles mockingly. A curious feeling somewhere between relief, resentment and embarrassment is quickly replaced by a recurring image. When I die, it will not be my life which flashes before my eyes, but Mrs P.'s bowel, all twenty feet of it. And it will not flash, but glide majestically, enabling me to examine it all in painful detail. It will look entirely normal.

This daydream fades as I realise that Mrs P. is animatedly informing me that her gastrointestinal tract continues to make her life hell. This, at least, we have in common. Her face tells a different story: the fear which I instilled on her previous visit has evaporated. She is confident, adamant and lively again. I ponder on my recent preoccupation with Mrs P. and her treacherous rectum. In the past, I have always accepted missed diagnoses as bad luck, an inevitable risk of General Practice. As a result, ensuing self-reproach has always been kept in proportion. But with Mrs P., I experienced such anguish: this because we have developed a special, symbiotic relationship over the years. Our consultations exist on a unique, mutually satisfying plane, and it occurs to me that I broke some unwritten rules during her last visit. Mrs P.'s bowel, as I should know by now, requires aural rather than surgical attention.

I relax, my thoughts again meander; I revel in the space which Mrs P.'s white noise of complaint permits me. In my mind, an imaginary conversation takes place.

Well, Mrs P., the results have come through and it's as I thought.

What is it doctor?

I adopt my best information-imparting voice, designed to display authority without creating anxiety. It inevitably fails on both counts. 'You have the Irritable Bowel Syndrome.'

'Oh no, doctor, it can't just be that.' Mrs P. is insulted. 'It can't be an irritable bowel, it's much too severe. Furious bowel, at least.'

I return to the reality of the surgery from my reverie, noticing that she has paused for breath. We all allow ourselves the luxury of a smile, a belly smile: myself, the devil on my shoulder, and Mrs P. Then she rambles on, my mind wanders and we are back in familiar territory. I realise that she does as much for me as I do for her and I love her for it. I love her, though I still hate her guts.

KEITH HOPCROFT
Basildon

The Doctor's Song

(Tune: *British Grenadiers*)

Some talk of hepatitis and some of Crohn's disease,
Of ulcerative colitis, of piles and such as these,
But there's a gut disorder makes doctors throw in the towel
With a rum tum tum tum tum tum, it's the irritable bowel.

For diverticulosis and peptic ulcer too,
Once make the diagnosis, you know just what to do
But who can name a remedy, with confident avowal,
With a rum tum tum tum tum tum, for the irritable bowel?

We try not to alarm them, we fill them up with bran,
We tell them it won't harm them – to endure it if they can,
But if there's one case where patients lay their symptoms on
    with a trowel,
With a rum tum tum tum tum tum, it's the irritable bowel.

MARIE CAMPKIN
London

5
Advice to Patients

Our doctors ... eat the melon and drink the new wine
while they keep their patients tied down to syrups and
slops

MICHEL DE MONTAIGNE[4]
1533–1592

H *ealthy eating is, of course, important and a high residue – or*
high refuse – diet, as a candidate in the PLAB examination for
overseas doctors wrote, can prevent disorders of the colon such as irrit-
able colon, cancer and diverticulosis. But patients can easily be
deprived of the pleasures of the table unnecessarily, partly because of
the myths and traditions that label certain foods as indigestible and
partly due to the lack of controlled trials; diets, like drugs, should be
subjected to these. Allergy, for example, so often lies in the mind
rather than the gastric mucosa.

'The pleasures of the table are of all times and all ages, of every coun-
try and of every day; they go hand in hand with all other pleasures,
outlast them and, in the end, console us for their loss', wrote Jean Bril-
lat-Savarin, advocate and gastronome, in his book The Physiology
of Taste or Meditation on Transcendental Gastronomy *written*
in 1825. One distraught general practitioner (a man of charm who
otherwise never used violent language) said to a woman who was
obsessed with what she ate 'Eat what the hell you like'. Perhaps this
wise council should be proferred more often. Many should be encour-
aged to abandon themselves to the pleasures of the table: fresh instead
of stale bread and strong instead of weak tea (in contrast to the advice
on some diet sheets), and even such delicacies protrayed by Brillat-
Savarin as 'the bliss of chicken fricasse', 'the suavity of vanilla merin-
gue', 'the savoury eel', and the 'lordly lobster'.[5]

Eating My Own Words

'D'you mean to tell me that after a bavarian meal and a ghastlyscope you still don't know what's wrong with him?' Mrs Armitage looked forlornly at her son.

I decided to appeal to the stricken victim directly. 'Wayne, the hospital can't find any serious cause for your stomach pains, so it's most likely some sort of simple gastritis. Other than the tablets you're already taking the answer lies in what we in the trade call "general measures". For a start it doesn't help that you're twenty-two stone ...'

'All our family are big-boned', interjected Mrs A. I dismissed this objection with a wave of my hand. 'And you've really got to cut down on all that junk food you're getting yourself around. Look at me, a picture of health, and I've never been in a burger bar in my life!' Balint would have been proud. I had put the argument cogently, cohesively, and in terms the patient could understand.

Wayne looked at me with the sullenness right and proper to a cove of barely twenty summers, reached within his flowing

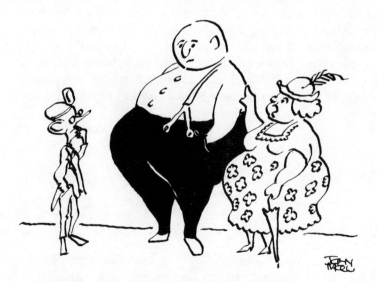

All our family are big boned

locks, and pulled his Walkman headset down over his neck. 'You say something, Doc?' 'Nothing important, Wayne,' I sighed. 'Just keep taking the tablets.'

I ushered the patient and his still-protesting mother out of the surgery, slightly guilty that I had not told them the whole truth. No man with children can escape burger bars forever, but I do try to restrict my visits to biennial celebrations of my offsprings' birthdays.

As luck would have it, just such an occasion presented itself the following week, and with the strength of ten wild horses my progeny dragged me over the threshold of the local fast-food emporium. I strode manfully up to the counter. 'Two Flatusburgers, one Waterbrash Special, and three boxes of what you laughingly describe as French fries, please.'

'Well, well, Doctor, fancy seeing you here!' The peroxide highlights of the heavily lacquered coiffure should have signalled danger a mile off, but I was too engrossed in the full horror of the epicurean fate that was to befall me. 'Mrs Armitage? What are you doing here?' 'I work here, Doctor. Have done for months. Now what was it you wanted? Two Flatusburgers ...'

'Ha! Me? Burgers? No!' I laughed. 'Never touch 'em. Just a cup of coffee, please.' I slunk away and sent the kids up for the burgers, hoping Mrs A. wouldn't notice the family resemblance. That night, all attempts to drift into the arms of Morpheus were thwarted, as waves of oesophageal reflux swept through me. Which goes to prove that your sins will not only find you out, they also have a habit of repeating themselves.

LAURENCE KNOTT
Enfield

In For Trouble?

M iss G. wants another diet. Or some slimming pills. Or the operation that was on the telly last night. Or an injection of brown fat. Or her own fat sucking away.

Miss G. is eighteen stone and rising. She never eats a thing, except lettuce leaves and cottage cheese. She overflows the chair in front of me. She has tried the Scarsdale diet, made a pilgrimage to Cambridge and constructed an F-Plan. She has tried grapefruit before the cottage cheese and papaya afterwards. She has steered clear of Ayds, because of the government campaign. Her weekly diet magazines are full of young, slim and attractive ladies, who have to be photographed full-frontal or the camera misses them. Doctor, some of it must be water retention. (But the diuretics given in a moment of weakness by Another Person did not help.) The articles tell her to consult her GP before taking up any new forms of exercise. She wants to run a marathon, as all the runners are ultra-thin.

Miss G., I wish I had the answer. We could wire your teeth, staple your stomach, excise your bowel, blow balloons up in your intestines, or vacuum-clean the fat away. The feminists say you still would not be happy. You are cocooned in fat because of insecurity and lack of confidence. You say you want to be thin. I won't prescribe the pills. Here is a high-fibre diet sheet that will not work either, but at least your bowels will!

JILL THISTLETHWAITE
Luddendon

Eat and Drink Less, Old Chap

I n the early evening, two men sat near the fire of the quiet village pub, tending their pints.

'You know,' started the less creased-looking of the pair. 'I hate this time of year, Tom. It's the dregs of Winter and everyone is so glum.'

'Probably half of my patients at the moment are suffering primarily from the season,' agreed Tom, looking up from the sheer interest of trying to remove the froth from the sides of his glass without disturbing the liquid it contained. His companion, Bill, was showing the signs of mental activity. 'Today, I think I'd seen about four of them already, when an old chap came in and sat down and didn't even have an excuse,' he said, 'so I gave him the lecture – the timeless one about eating less, drinking less, exercising more.' He stopped, ruefully dissecting his beer mat.

'Sounds to me like your nerve has finally broken, trying to lecture to an old chap about healthy living,' Tom suggested wryly. 'Still, a lot of them could do a lot worse than to watch their weight a bit more: I'm sure that's part of the reason for the seasonal depression – unfitness, that is.'

'But they won't listen to logic will they, so they'll all be back again next year and the year after,' added Bill. Tom nodded his agreement and consulted his watch. 'Drink up,' he said, 'I think we deserve another.' 'We certainly do,' agreed Bill vehemently. 'I don't think I could face the walk home yet, anyway.' 'Too true,' said Tom, standing up with a groan and tucking his shirt in below his pendulous abdomen.

SAUL MILLER
Cardiff

I *would prescribe a high refuse diet—an examination candidate's answer.*

6
Wind and Other Unsavoury Matters

And then I did a thing will make you laugh,
For as he neared me, by some divine mishap
My wind exploded like a thunder clap,
I guess the God was awfully disgusted.
No, but Iaso blushed a rosy red
And Panacea turned away her head
Holding her nose: my wind's not frankincense

ARISTOPHANES
445–*c.* 380 BC[6]

T he expulsion of flatus is an ancient source of humour as is shown
by the above quotation from Aristophanes' comedy **The Plutus**.
But still it is considered by patients to be a sign of indigestion, es-
pecially if the belch is flavoured by aromatic odours from a meal. The
patient mistakenly diagnoses discomfort as due to wind and tries to
disperse it by eructation. This results in swallowing of air, for a gulp
usually precedes belching: the air merely distends the oesophagus or,
with repeated efforts, is forced into the stomach. Many think that this
'wind' which they belch is due to fermentation in the stomach – a sort
of marsh gas generated because what they eat is not digesting properly.
Actually this can happen – though rarely – in pyloric stenosis: food
may remain in the stomach for 24 hours or more and undergoes bac-
terial decomposition which produces hydrogen or methane – an eruc-
tation at the moment of lightening a cigarette has resulted in an
inflammable belch causing a slight burn on the nose, and, in another
case, alarm was caused when it occurred in the darkness of a cinema.
Belching, usually just a nervous habit, can be a nuisance and irritate
others, such as the spouse, as illustrated by 'A Breath of Air' (see
Chapter 10) and by the following story:

Belching Affects Others

Dr Jones's outpatient clinic always remains crowded. Maybe he is very popular. Maybe more gastrointestinal problems are prevalent. Maybe he is slow, like a psychiatrist who takes much longer to take a history, asking many intimate questions. His clinic always goes beyond time. So what? Actually, this is relevant. A particular patient, let us call him Mr X. I can't give his real name or he will see his solicitor for libel. Don't ask about Dr Jones, as I must assure you he is not real either. But, believe me, the story is real, or at least what I am going to say. Back to Mr X: 5'6", blond hair, blue eyes, pale complexion, anxious, trying to play with his fingers, biting his lips and finger-nails; not very smartly dressed. Kept burping wind and kept saying 'beg your pardon'. Who pardons anyway? Suppose one does not pardon, can you stop burping or can you go on burping without taking notice of others? I

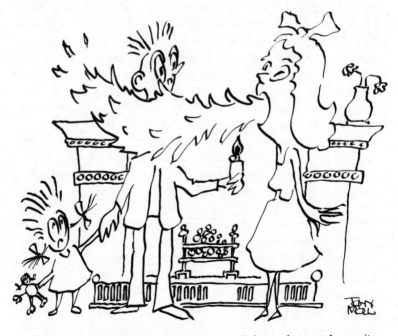

The inflammable belch ignited by a cigarette lighter—fortunately a rarity

thought he could just keep a hand-written notice to say 'pardon me' and point to it every time he burped or say once loudly 'Pardon me and I am sorry I can't stop burping. Not my fault. Dr Jones won't cure me'.

I could hear whispers. Some were annoyed. Some felt sorry for him. I thought, it is disgusting that he can't stop burping. I felt that he could ask for cold water or suck or chew antacid tablets; it was incredible, and I was very concerned. Honestly speaking, I was so concerned that I thought I might suggest something. But you won't believe me, I started hiccups at this moment. Didn't I say incredible? Yes, it was a coincidence and I couldn't stop. One thing was different: I kept saying 'I am sorry, after each hiccup', not 'beg your pardon'. Well, again it is not important. Then a funny thing happened; I got up to go, as I thought I was called, but soon realised that I was the wrong person. You get amnesia if you are in deep thought. That minishock stopped my hiccups. But Mr X still kept burping . . .

R.P. YADAVA
Stoke-on-Trent

Thesis on 'The Bowel Sounds with tape recordings of borborygmi and a demonstration gramophone record.' The degree of CH.M. was awarded to J.M. Mynors by the University of Birmingham in 1963

Whereas belching is acceptable and even encouraged in some cultures — being an indication of approval for the food of one's hostess, wind expelled through the lower orifice is seldom appreciated in any company; yet after an operation, it is a cardinal sign that the patient's bowel is recovering function. Communication then is a problem: the intelligent patient may respond to the enquiry as to whether he or she

has expelled flatus per rectum, or passed wind through the back pass-
age, but the farm labourer or navvy, for example, who is semicon-
scious and recovering from a major abdominal operation is better
approached with the question 'Can you fart?' But unfortunately brief
onomatopoeic Anglo-Saxon words like pee and fart are not in current
usage and are not used in a hospital ward. However, there is nothing
inherently bad in these and, as Fritz Spiegl wrote,[7] *'rude' words are*
rude and ugly only by habit and repute; indeed 'arse' was the standard
polite word for tail in the seventeenth century – even in the law courts.
So it was with other four-letter words. John Aubrey recounted the sad
tale of the Earl of Oxford who 'making of his low obeisance to Queen
Elizabeth, happened to let a fart, at which he was so abashed and
ashamed that he went to travell, 7 yeares. On his return the Queen
welcomed him home, and sayd, My Lord, I had forgot the Fart'.[8]
Aubrey was a writer who loved sensational gossip and the Earl did
seem to overreact but the word must have been in common use at that
time.

The natural function of defaecation has not always been regarded
with disgust and shame. Louis XIV received his courtiers as he sat on
a 'chaise percée' feeling in no way embarrassed that he was relieving
himself publicly. But matters associated with the function of the lower
gut are now an unsavoury topic for genteel conversation. Hence the
euphemisms for the watercloset; powder room, or 'would you like to
wash your hands?' – and many loos are bare undecorated chilly places
with nothing to gaze at on the walls or door. Yet everyone has to spend
time there and the costive much longer. Little attention is given to
public 'conveniences' optimistically called 'Ladies' and 'Gentlemen';
and equality does not exist, for ladies are at a pecuniary disadvantage.

A Penny for Your Thoughts

The digestive system is a splendid institution. What pleasure arouses – appetite, the consideration of the thought of
intake, the twitching nose, the moistening of lips, the saliva-
tory anticipation – then the senses at rest, the infinite realms of
converse as the gastric nerves respond to soothing, possibly

the words of love, as are the heart and stomach not closely linked, both in poetry and blood supply? Alas, the end result may not always be so happy.

In former days, gargantuan intake assumed painful progress and delayed output. Who as an infant has not been seated on a small round disc, promised the sugared biscuit if 'good', and the fell dark draught if 'bad'? Or is life now better harnessed with disposables and congratulations? Read the words of Samuel Pepys and his fellows – of the green Bile, the Stone – or of Jane Welsh Carlyle, and that family essential, the Blue Pill.

We come now to what are described as 'toilet facilities'. In one northern capital an adjunct for gentlemen was established in the High Street, frequently attended by the city council. One charitably suggested to the well-known attendant present year in, year out, that he should take a holiday. On calling there for relief the next week, he found that gentleman in a handsome new jersey.

'You should be on holiday,' he exploded.

'Yes, sir, but you said I could have it at my own convenience,' was the reply.

Gentlemen have always been favoured in these haunts, which are far more readily available than those for ladies. Gentlemen are also more fortunate when sick, retiring beneath the covers with receptacle. Ladies must ring for Nurse, and perch.

During the last century the ladies of pleasure of Regent Street descended neatly within their crinolines in the open air. The ladies of the high Andes, who resemble small triangular tea-cosies, still sink to the ground in a circle of petticoats, and pass on.

For a long time, ladies of the peerage were forbidden entry to the House of Lords despite their primacy, as there was nowhere for their periodic comfort. (There is reasonable accommodation now, with the added amenity of a large hand-mirror, chained to the wall. Is this asset also available to male Peers?)

In Mexico City, penniless owing to a temporarily confiscated passport on a long day between planes from Australia to Peru, and suffering from a native fruit drink of doubtful content, two doors presented CABALLEROS and SEÑORAS. On hurried entry a stout moustached female insisted on remuneration, which was unavailable. Compulsory occupation resulted in loud cries and recriminations.

Escaping cowed, a secondary arrangement was perceived behind a row of bootblacks, a drop in the social scale, but gratis. Here were found HOMBRES and DAMAS. The doors reached from neck to knees, but were unguarded. For conditions threatening dysentry, this should receive recognition from the Mexican government.

At one stage turnstiles were introduced to female conveniences, which resulted in impaction to the pregnant. A survey of these obstructions was conducted by the Medical Women's Federation who, unsung, brought about their removal. There still remain reduced specimens that might impact a dwarf, but there is a hole to crawl through.

The fact remains that ladies are at a post-digestive disadvantage. Should they forego the pleasures of eating, perhaps? What a missed opportunity for the present government – free female pissoires will ensure 50% national support, even without the need to voting and, who knows, perhaps a seat in the cabinet?

CYSTIA

Euphemisms for a Water-closet

Lavatory (a wash basin)

Toilet (cloth cover for a dressing table)

Loo

Privy

The House of Office

The Necessarium

'I have finally kum to the konklusion, that a good
reliable sett ov bowels iz wurth more tu a man, then
enny quantity ov brains.'

JOSH BILLINGS
1818–1885[9]

*The bowels, though not a subject to discuss at a bridge party, have been
a preoccupation with individuals – especially in the past. Patients
have taken a special interest, describing their bowels as 'respectable,
beautiful or stubborn' and felt that they understood their bowels better
than anyone else possibly could – an opinion Britons seldom extended
to other organs, like the liver.*

Bowels as a Hobby

The French may love their livers, but it's we Brits who are
besotted by our bowels. Perhaps this is *the* British disease.
Many a matronly English Rose would blush at the very
thought of describing other 'down below' diseases to her doctor, but she'll wax lyrical when asked about 'trouble with the
bowels'. 'Trouble' is invariably synonymous with constipation, which the dictionary defines as 'difficult or infrequent
defaecation'. What is difficult or infrequent to the patient is
seldom regarded as either by their practitioner.

Getting potty about her botty is not the patient's fault. It's
probably an inherited disease. You certainly catch it from your
Victorian parents, who've instilled the belief in daily defaecation as the only sure route to both spiritual and bodily purity.
Medical professionals are not immune. Some older psychiatric
nurses remain convinced that trouble up top invariably begins
in the bottom. On general hospital wards the staff lovingly
record the toilet trips of each of their patients in the ward
'bowel book', though I am aware of no doctor ever perusing
these pages. Perhaps this record of the daily 'doings' of the

occasional celebrity patient may be of future interest to the *News of the World*.

Bran and other fashionable food fads have made 'botty blues' trendy, lowering the age range of complainants and raising our surgery attendance statistics. For some sufferers, bowels are a hobby to be discussed with anyone vaguely medical from chiropodist to neurologist, though the loudest complainers of constant colonic congestion are rarely those most at risk of the much-feared 'stoppage'. One lady patient whose empty cavernous nether regions I have explored with a frequency sufficient to arouse the suspicions of the GMC complains of a period of absolute constipation which, were it found to be true, would certainly qualify for the Guiness Book of Records.

This is not to belittle true constipation, which can be a painful and distressing condition, occasionally presenting as a medical emergency. Too much toiling on the toilet is distinctly unhealthy – it is not unusual for last gasps to be taken in the smallest room. True constipation in no way accounts for the prolific national consumption of purgatives. Long-term laxative abuse becomes an addiction, which can parodoxically cause constipation. Millions of geriatric guts prohibit peristalsis until kick-started by a daily fix of aperient. Hospital is the worst place to kick this habit. It's probably where you got hooked. Lack of privacy, strange plumbing and immobility rarely leave hospital patients flushed with success. Not to worry! Friendly pushers dressed as nurses will happily supply (without charge) copious quantities of the NHS-favoured liquid laxative. Rumour has it that this purgative panacea is now delivered to larger hospitals in tankers.

JOHN SQUIRE
Ilkley

Young patients today discuss other topics than their bowels.

The Ins and Outs of General Practice: Outward Bound?

Mrs G. wants another house call. She has trouble with her bowels – again. Every one of those old people's flats is occupied by an ageing lady who wants to set her clock by the movements of her colon. If she has not performed by 10 a.m. there is panic and despair. My own gut-feeling is more likely to be spasmodic in frustration. I carry micro-enemas, borrowed from the district nurse's box of tricks; so useful for the weekend emergency blockage when I cannot stomach another manual removal. I nod sympathetically at the tales of bloating tummies, ignore the several brands of self-administered laxatives and decide that trying to change the thought processes of a lifetime is no match for the daily fix of senna.

In my mind's eye I conjure up a picture of hundreds of Edwardian mamas impressing on their offspring the purgative values of a morning motion. The large brown medicine bottle, full of an evil-tasting elixir, awaits the child who neglects his duty.

The younger patients seem embarrassed to discuss the nature of their evacuations. They will talk for what seems like hours, and quite explicitly, on sex and drugs and contraception. Toilet habits are private. Vaginal examinations, though unwelcome, appear more natural than the dreaded rectal exploration.

Mrs D. likes to describe her toilet triumphs to this reluctant audience of one. She attends the surgery cheerfully on her good days. Yes, she had performed well this morning, the world is a wonderful place. On her bad days, it takes the promise of a litre of lactulose to bring a smile to her lips and a spring to her gait. Every year, while the unions fight it out for a satisfactory rise, Mrs S. has her annual senna increment to keep things ticking over as before. She has had so much medicine over the decades that her bowels are now completely free of any autonomic control. Her senna load is increasing exponentially with time.

It is hard to understand the real anguish of these patients. As a full-of-fibre person myself, once a day is rarely enough. Bran works a treat for me, but it only makes the old ladies more costive and crotchety.

But what do I do about Mrs R.? She goes regularly, but forgets her toilet trips as her memory is failing. Yet she remembers well her lovely mother with the large brown bottle and the silver table spoon.

Anyway, Mrs G. wants another house call. The suppositories worked rather too well and she has been twice this morning and that can't be right . . . can it doctor?

JILL THISTLETHWAITE
Luddendon

A European interest is included in the two next contributions.

Language – Onomatopoeia and the Bowels

Do you remember the one about the businessman who wanted a crash course in Japanese? You just have to sound cold, constipated and querulous all at the same time . . . and therein lies the problem – there are numerous stories of that type but they only exist in the oral tradition because there are no written equivalents to the sounds they rely on to make us laugh. The centre-piece of that story lies in the enunciation of a sound made by leakage of air through the larynx whilst increasing the intra-abdominal pressure to . . . well anyway, you know what I mean.

I recall as a junior doctor fretting over whether or not a woman was fully dilated towards the end of her protracted labour. The midwife, wordly wise as ever, said 'She'll tell you when she's ready' and sure enough, within half an hour we heard a sound best described as 'uuuuuuuunnnnnnnhhhh'. But there again, it's not really the right spelling, is it? How many of us have tried to describe to our two-year-olds what it feels like 'when you want a pooh' and failed, a look of disbelief on our loved ones'. faces as we strain away. This great language, which from Chaucer to Sid James has been preoccupied with the humour of the bowels and the apparatus connected with them, has failed to evolve appropriate sounds to describe a number of everyday physiological (and sometimes pathological) functions. Medical education, so skilled in the use of onomatopoeia in cardiology, has failed in respect to gastro-enterology. (Now, let's listen to her as she passes a motion here – does it go 'plop' or is it more of a 'thphelch' – no madam, don't worry about our medical jargon.)

Our public has, in some fields however, not been so coy. A review of the literature produces a wealth of dialect sounds and words. I would select guff, belch and rift as shining examples; there are numerous others, some imaginative, some plain boastful, but none quite *le mot juste*.

The European medical establishment has not let us down and there are powerful lessons to be learnt from them. We should not be surprised, for these are the countries where the suppository is king. The French, bless them, quite liked vomit but because they won't pronounce their endings it wasn't nearly as effective, so they settled for the more evocative *le vomissure* and if you stress all the syllables it's almost as good as Winston, or Hughie and Ruth. But the greatest feat of language belongs to the Spanish who, not satisfied with constipation (or even *la constipation*), use the masterly *estrenimiento* which, enunciated clearly and loudly is more effective than tabs senna, take two at night. *Ole!*

ANDREW PROCTER
Bury

Euro Dung

'I'm supposed to show you this.' The respectable, well-spoken man produced, with not inconsiderable pride, a card saying that he was in contact with human sewage.

It is my custom to see all my new patients as they register. After a preliminary chat about everyday things, I discovered that this middle-aged man worked at the airport.

'We get sewage from all over the world,' he explained. All doctors have more than a hint of nosiness. I was becoming intrigued. 'I may have to handle this material sometimes,' he further tempted.

My mind raced ahead of him. Perhaps it was one of those days when right brain was dominating left. Imagination was out-pacing logic.

My mind was conjuring up visions of huge sealed containers, laden with raw sewage. I could visualise, hear, almost smell the sewage slopping and slurping around.

Perhaps he had to inspect the contents. Perhaps he had to decide which processing plant would be best suited to a particular batch. Perhaps there were different texture and types. Perhaps some needed urgent attention. Perhaps some needed specialised refinement.

The whole scheme seemed perfectly reasonable. I had heard that Britain was accepting nuclear waste from all over Europe for processing and detoxification. Perhaps the same applied to processing the waste products of the bowels of half of Europe.

We all know about wine lakes and butter mountains. Perhaps this was Euro dung – a sort of bilge bulge.

My respect for this man was growing by the minute. A very unpleasant, even dangerous job. But obviously very necessary for Britain's trade balance.

Unfortunately he elaborated further on his story by telling me that he was a cleaner in the airport toilets. Can't be right all the time!

CHRISTOPHER J. BARRETT
Northwich

The state of the patient's stools provides an invaluable diagnostic aid for the doctor, particularly in cases of intestinal bleeding, malabsorption or colitis, but obtaining this information is fraught with difficulty: the patient may not have looked at his faeces or the nurse may have thrown them away without reporting on them.

Stool Gazing

This is a nebulous subject of atmosphere, motion and globular clusters; flat or round masses depending on your viewpoint or whether you have actually been lucky enough to have a reasonable look. How many of us slam down the loo seat without so much as a 'look back in anger' only to find the bottom has dropped out of our world or we sail off the edge later on? The ancient Greeks and Pythagorus, in their belief that the earth was flat, received support from observation; for example, the earth's shadow on the moon and the stars' motion relative to one's own position on the earth. When we perform that most private of functions any change from normality can be sensed, but without direct observation its significance can be seriously underestimated.

In the medical profession one is taught that observation comes first in all examinations, followed by palpation, percussion and finally auscultation. No doubt there are some enthusiasts who would attempt all four; however, descriptions more attributable to pastry-making or play-dough are unlikely to provide more information than a quick look and sniff. Certainly I have yet to hear anything recognisable using even the most powerful electronic stethoscope. I doubt if the dumbest worm or parasite would dare slither or scratch in a characteristic way, and fizzing or bubbling even after the hottest curry isn't usual. It would be of more value to put the stethoscope to the WC door and recognise the agonising squeal and sharp intake of breath of a severe shortage of fibre and probable anal fissure, or the gentle pitter-patter of a bitter man's bottom.

Returning to our main subject of direct observation, before you all go out and buy stethoscopes, pH kits and thermometers. Unfortunately when I qualified, matron's stool round on the ward each morning was already a thing of the past. Therefore, as for most students and housemen, the art of stool gazing for me remained mainly self-taught. It was during these first years in medicine that I decided that it would be much better for patients and even non-patients to learn this themselves. There would be a major saving on air freshener (and therefore the ozone layer), smelling salts and 'Kwells' in hospital clinics and GP's surgeries. How much better it would be to see an immediate smile of understanding on Mrs Jones' face when asked about black motion instead of a quizzical frown as she remembers seeing the 'Jackson Five' on their last UK tour.

In our wisdom we have made culinary descriptions for the most unsavoury stools. The cranberry jelly stool for a child with intussusception, peas and carrot stool of innocent toddler diarrhoea, rice-water stool of cholera, all allow people to describe what they see without feeling nauseous. We should encourage people to also recognise the silver stool of cancer of the pancreas, the sticky fatty floating stool of malabsorption, the rabbit pellet or ribbon-like stool of irritable bowel, and as many others as we can think of. Instead of hearing 'but I never look, doctor', think how helpful it would be to immediately be presented with a full and recognisable description. Herschel pioneered and catalogued 2500 star clusters and nebulae in his time; I don't expect us to be able to describe as many different stools, or stool gazing to become like reading tea leaves. However, 'look before you flush' would be a useful slogan to spread far and wide.

J.G. MELLOR
Cottingham

All in the Mind

D r Boris Charles put aside his *Which Fishing Rod?* report to greet the familiar, untidy figure entering the room.

'Morning, Doc,' said Gordon, untoggling his duffle coat and rummaging in his Tesco bag. 'I want this analysed, please.' He produced a large coffee-jar, precariously close to over-flowing with a semi-formed, mahogany coloured, and, judging by the condensation, fresh faecal specimen.

'Know what's in there?' asked Gordon furtively. 'Well,' whispered Dr Charles in reply, 'this is what we doctors call a turd.' Gordon roared with laughter and thumped the desk, millimetres from the offending container. 'Aye. And I want it analysed. For poison.' 'Any particular poison, Gordon? They have to know what to aim for, you know.' 'Aye, I've been doing some research.' He delved again into his carrier bag and unearthed a tattered square of paper. It read:

MON 21th FEB.

BURNING in OESOPAGUS. As redhot POKER!

CRAMPS. Peripatetic. V. severe. As if small int.
fed thro mangle.

DIAREHOA. *BURNS* (ow). Pellets of undigested
matter 1·5 cm. diameter, texture of cooked BANANA.

'So what do you suspect?' interrupted Dr Charles. 'Ah. The short-list.' Gordon fumbled again in his filing system 'Here we are.'

SUSPECTED POISONS & SOURCES —

1.   White oxide of ARSENIC. (toothpaste cap
been disturbed again)
2.   Roots of white HELLEBORE (suspicious
fragments in HAGGIS & CHIPS from
MACDOUGALL'S, 19 Feb.)
3.   Extract of Bitter Cucumber COLOCYNTHIS
(pickled gherkin served with 2)
4.   Strontium 90 EGG CUSTARD (Muriel's?)

'You should be able to detect the strontium easily.' 'Yes, I'll alert the lab.' 'Oh, I nearly forgot. Here's another specimen that might help you.'

Dr Charles shuddered in anticipation, but this time Gordon displayed a brown paper bag, inside which was a plastic sandwich box housing another paper bag, which in turn contained an orange. Gordon slowly rotated it to reveal an Elastoplast adherent to its equatorial zone.

'Know what this is?' 'Er, a radio transmitter?' 'Now, don't joke with me, Doc, this is serious.' 'All right, it's an orange.' 'Know what's inside it?' 'Orange juice?' Gordon yanked off the Elastoplast with a flourish. 'Look!' Dr Charles looked. 'There! See it now?' said Gordon testily, jabbing his finger at the fruit. 'No.' 'A puncture site, see? Been injected with poison.' He looked gravely at the doctor. 'You want it analysed.' 'I want it analysed.'

Jessie the receptionist knew the routine. Gordon, being impervious to conventional ends-of-consultation hints, was being gently escorted to the door by Dr Charles, 'Yes, Gordon, come back next Monday and we'll have some results.'

The next patient – in this instance Miss Stirling (she of church organ fame) – was shown deftly into the consulting room to prevent one of Gordon's U-turns.

Dr Charles duly entered, relieved to have completed his weekly test of psychiatric expertise. 'Why, Miss Stirling! You look awful!' Indeed she did. Beads of sweat accumulated on her cold, white brow. Her jaw quivered, and her eyes focused glassily on a large coffee jar on the desk.

ALAN DAVIS
St Austell

Bowel problems, whether constipation or diarrhoea, are humiliating though fortunately the anus – called the sentinel of social security – usually functions normally and protects from the disasters of incontinence.

7
Diagnostic Dilemmas

Errors in judgement must occur in the practice of an art
which consists largely in balancing probabilities

WILLIAM OSLER
1849 – 1919[10]

Technological advances in medicine have been remarkable since William Osler said this but, in many specialities, diagnosis is still an art rather than an exact science. Hence, medicine can be the most humiliating of all the professions, for in spite of a conscientious attention to every detail of a patient's problem, failures, as well as successes in diagnosis can occur.*

Tracey Lee's Tummy Pain

It was half an hour before the close of evening surgery, that perilous gloaming during which patients rush up with their problems to avoid calling the doctor out at night. Mrs Lee appeared at the reception desk with Tracey, aged seven, who looked a little dazed.

'She's complaining of tummy pain,' said Mrs Lee, 'and she's been sick and dizzy. She's not herself. You know we never trouble you unless it's absolutely necessary.'

The last statement was blatantly untrue. All the Lee tribe had records as thick as family bibles. Dr Jane Swift was the duty doctor for the evening and she agreed to see Tracey at once. 'How long have you had the pain, Tracey,' she asked. Tracey looked dumbly at her mother and didn't answer. 'Since she came home from school, doctor,' prompted her mother. Jane noticed that Tracey was swaying slightly in her seat and appeared to be about to fall to floor. Mrs Lee was sure it was appendicitis.

The little girl certainly looked unwell. She was flushed and seemed to be 'not with it'. The pain was over the stomach, but gentle probing did not cause tenderness. In fact, Tracey seemed to be about to go off to sleep on the examination couch. The practice was weathering a meningitis scare at the time. Jane Swift had only been a GP for three years and had never seen a case except in hospital, but every parent in the town was on a short fuse because there had been a teenager with it in the local hospital. Jane checked Tracey's neck carefully for signs of stiffness and searched meticulously for the blotchy skin haemorrhages which are characteristic of the disease. Nothing came to light.

Was it diabetes, perhaps? Abdominal pain is a common feature in childhood diabetic pre-coma and Tracey was certainly drowsy.

'Has she been thirsty and going to the loo more than usual?' Jane asked Mrs Lee. There was a negative response. 'Breathe out,' she told Tracey and lowered her head close to the young patient's mouth. Was that acetone – a sign of diabetes after all? No, surely it was something much commoner and easy to recognise, especially as Jane had unpleasant memories of Saturday night as a casualty officer.

'What have you been drinking, Tracey?' enquired she with a suspicious twinkle in her eyes, 'and how much?' 'I only had four glasses of Grandad's home-made wine'; the reply was now definitely slurred.

Mrs Lee was highly embarrassed. 'Fancy a daughter of mine drunk and only seven,' she flustered.

Except for a slight hangover, Tracey was none the worse for her experience after a good night's sleep and Jane had a marvellous story to tell at lunch in the postgraduate centre. Grandad is now making ginger beer.

JOHN WOODWARD
Sidcup

(A physician colleague was just leaving a house where he had consulted with a GP about an infant in coma – having failed to make a diagnosis and about to fix admission to hospital – when he spotted a

large empty bottle labelled 'Gripe Water'. It, like many prescriptions for this, contained a miniscule quantity of alcohol; but the parents had been desperate in trying to quieten the crying baby, which had drunk the entire bottle and was in an alcoholic coma. Ed.)

Wart a Mistake

You know how it is when you have gained experience. You don't have to spend all that precious time turning people on their left-hand side or examining neck veins, tapping out the borders of the heart and so on. Be selective! Of course, you've got to do it when these Trainees are around, but, thank God, when they're able to work on their own, you can get on easily without the danger of 'burn-out'.

So it was with relief that I got the Trainee doing his own surgery, and no doubt he was glad to get away from me. In any case, I was shortly going on holiday, and had a lot to get through. Miss Oxley was my first patient and I hadn't seen her for a while, but I knew her well as an amiable self-neglecting spinster, who could not do enough for her half-dozen cats.

When she came in, she was as blue as a whinberry. Breathless too. She sat down with difficulty, summoned all her faded charm, and pointed at a wart on her nose. 'I should like to have this removed', she said. 'Spoiling your beauty, is it?' I asked with medical irony. She must have been surprised when I looked instead at her ankles! Underneath the wrinkled and dirty old stocks were the best example of bilateral ankle oedema you could wish to see. Here, if ever there was one, was a case of severe congestive cardiac failure. A few hurried routine question followed. Had she had a sudden attack of weakness, shortness of breath, or pain in the chest? 'Not really,' she replied, but she admitted that she had put on a lot of weight over the past few months, and found getting about more difficult. 'Aha,' I exclaimed in one of those rare moments of supreme confidence when you have hit the diagnostic nail on the head, 'we shall soon have you feeling loads better!'

I explained, even though she appeared inattentive, that her heart was under a lot of strain, and not pumping properly – failing, in fact. I was going away in a couple of days, but would call round first thing in the morning, as I passed her house on my way in, and would give her an injection. 'You'll have to stay indoors for a few hours' I explained, 'because you'll pass gallons of water, after which you'll feel tons better.' This was such a good case that I toyed with the idea of getting the Trainee in to see her. On the other hand, there wasn't much to learn from it, being so obvious, and I didn't want to get held up, nor start that interminable coming and going that sometimes happens. No! I would tell him about it when we had our next meeting. 'Alright, Miss Oxley. Thank goodness you came. I'll see you tomorrow!' That's the way to terminate a consultation, I told myself. No loose edges; an accurate diagnosis, the indicated treatment to be given in adequate dosage. What a pity I couldn't show the Trainee. But never mind. Meanwhile, Miss Oxley had wandered to the door. Her hand had grasped the handle. I was looking to see who would be the next patient, when she said 'What about this wart on my nose, doctor?' Well, you know how it is these days – the minor complaint as a passport to see the doctor about something more serious and occult. The look on Miss Oxley's face suggested that the gross cardiac failure was immaterial, and I had misjudged the real reason for her visit. 'We'll discuss that when I see you tomorrow, Miss Oxley,' I said encouragingly, and she left.

Next morning I called at 8 a.m. at her house. Like Miss Oxley, the house had seen better days. One had to pick one's way about because saucers of cat food and stale milk were everywhere. The smell in the house was such that I did not want to stay. 'Let us go up to your bedroom, as I want to give you the injection here', I said, indicating the buttock area. She then led me to a bedroom, where a couple of cats lay in a bed long unmade or laundered. All my professional training was summoned to my aid as I surveyed the expanse of buttock I was about to inject. It never occurred to me that I had no chaperone, but recounting the story now I feel sure the GMC would temper justice with mercy. I gave the 100 mg frusemide without incident, and left her a dozen Slow K to take over the next two days.

Next day I telephoned, and learned there had been a marvellous result. The Trainee came in for his tutorial. 'General practice can be very satisfying,' I said to him. 'Here was this woman. . .' and I told him about the case, as if such things were a daily occurrence, noting, not without satisfaction, how he nodded with approval. Trainers need this sometimes. Anyway, it was now time to say goodbye to partners and receptionists, as we were off next day to foreign parts. Not, we always hoped, ever to have the experience of Dr Taylor as he descended the gangway at Algeria, feeling the warm sun and noting the jellabas and fez below him, when he felt a hand on his shoulder and turned. There was his prize 'neurotic' patient expressing his relief to see his doctor, for he had forgotten to pack his sleeping tablets! No, nothing like that happened.

We returned sunbaked, restored by the Kasbah, inspired by the great mosque, nourished by fruit and wine. It takes a few days to get back on the old wave-length. One has to adjust slowly, but partners and receptionists are kind. They ease you back gently. The Trainee, having formally asked if we had a good holiday, seemed somehow awkward. Poor chap, it's not all fun being young. 'Everything alright, John?' I asked. 'Yes, yes!' he responded. 'By the way, Mrs Harper wants to see you.' 'OK,' I said, 'I expect she's going through the morning list with me.' 'You seem to have been away a long time, doctor,' said the chief receptionist. 'Thanks for your card, it looks a very interesting place.' 'Quite fascinating,' I answered. 'Oh! How is Miss Oxley?' 'She's very well now, and I've got her down for a follow-up visit. By the way, I've got a letter here for you about her.' 'Oh? I didn't refer her. Who's it from?' 'It's from Mr Clift, the Gynaecologist. The Trainee had to pay her an emergency visit, for abdominal pain.' 'Oh dear! Poor woman,' I responded, 'let me see the letter.' It read: 'Dear Keith, thank you very much for this very interesting patient. I have never seen such a big ovarian cyst in years. It weighed 17 lbs. Anyway, the removal was straightforward, and we'll send you the path report later. . . (my mind was going a bit blank) . . . Hoping you had a good holiday, best wishes, Ron.'

So, suntanned but not very relaxed, I made my way round to see Miss Oxley. She certainly looked a different shape and colour. I made my way in to the stale smell of cats. 'Sit down, doctor,' said Miss Oxley, indicating the filthy cat-laden sofa, and destroying in an instant memories of verdant paradise gardens and perfumed flowers represented on those beautiful patterned Islamic rugs! It was my role to be humble, my patient came first. She came and sat beside me, nursing two cats, while I had one crawling on my lap. 'Well, how are you, Miss Oxley? You look much better.' Miss Oxley allowed this comment to sink right in before she made her reply. It came rather suddenly and impulsively. She shifted right up close, put her arm through mine in a warm hug. As I looked closely at her face, her eyes were shining with admiration as she gushed: 'Doctor, you are a member of a wonderful profession!'

I don't quite know how I got out of that with the preservation of professional dignity. But I had now to face the Trainee, who obviously knew all that had happened. I knew the story would probably be all round the Trainers' group by now. What alternatives were open to me? I could ignore the matter, and maintain a false dignity. No. One could not live with that for another nine months. The right thing would be to point out that we continue learning, and that we learn best from our mistakes. On the other hand, this was not a mistake I should have made in the first place.

M. KEITH THOMPSON
Croydon

Misled by a Munchausen

Matthew Forbes had just come to the end of his introductory two months in general practice at the start of his three-year vocational training scheme at Handlebridge Hospital. He had applied to Handlebridge because he had heard that it was a good idea to train in the area in which one intended to settle as a partner in a practice. There were advantages, he had been told, in knowing the consultants and local family doctors.

The first of the four posts in Matthew's hospital rotation was in the hospital's Accident and Emergency department. He had been worried about this job because it was relatively unsupervised. Casualty officers, he knew, tended to be left alone to ward off the public who had a right to be seen although most of their troubles were minor conditions. 'You'll find,' he had been warned by his trainer Bill Adams, 'that they'll say they couldn't get an appointment to see their GP. Most of the things they'll bring to you won't really need a doctor at all. A junior first aid cadet could manage them without any problems.'

Matthew's first shift on duty, a Monday evening ending at 10 p.m., seemed to his relief to be passing without incident. He saw a child with a nosebleed, a welder with arc eye, two elderly ladies who had slipped – one of whom had a Colles fracture and the other a laceration on the shin. The ambulance brought in an RTA, a teenager who had been knocked off his bike and was reputed to have been unconscious for about ten minutes. Straightforward stuff, he thought to himself, not much different from a session in casualty at his medical school. All the same, he missed the comforting presence of his trainer, who usually did a surgery in an adjacent room. Bill Adams' practice had three partners and was situated in Yewbank, a village five miles from Handlebridge, where the pace of life was slow and everyone knew everyone else and people seemed to be normal. At Handlebridge, all was bustle and panic and nobody seemed to have time to chat to a new and rather frightened casualty SHO.

Just before Matthew came to the end of his first shift, the casualty staff nurse handed him a treatment card with details about another patient. 'This man's decidedly odd,' she said. 'He's complaining of tummy pain and rolling around in his chair, but his pulse and temperature are normal and so's his blood pressure. Will you see him?'

'Of course,' Matthew replied. 'Which cubicle is he in?' 'First on the left. Do you mind if I leave you by yourself? I've got a cut to sew up.'

The new patient, whose name was stated to be Patrick

McGlinty, was a thin worried-looking man in his early fifties. 'Good evening, Mr McGlinty,' Matthew began. 'Why have you come up to see us?'

'It's me pains, doctor'. The accent was neither Irish nor Scottish, but sounded like a mixture of London Dockland and the antipodes. 'They're bloody terrible and I can't stand them, any more.' 'Tell me about yourself', Matthew continued and, unprepared for the saga which followed, was soon settling back in his chair unable to get in a word to direct the case history into the familiar progression he had learned at medical school. 'Oh, I've had a lot of trouble with me guts, doctor. It all started when I was fifteen and they didn't take me appendix out before it perforated which left me with them adhesion things glueing up me insides. Then I had an ulcer in the army when I was twenty-three and they did two operations on that. I had me gall bladder out ten years later and then they had to cut me up to get at a stone in me kidneys. This time I think it's to do with an accident I had five years ago in the Congo, although the pain's different. I was on Major Smitecross-Crick's expedition and got thrown out of the canoe on some rapids and ruptured me spleen.'

Funny, thought Matthew to himself. I'm sure Smitecross-Crick went down the Congo before that. I remember he came to talk at school about it when I was in the sixth.

'They had to fly me home from Africa after taking the spleen out in a mission hospital,' McGlinty continued. 'That was me last operation, but this pain isn't quite the same as the ones I had after they did that. It's more in the centre and goes through to me back.'

The story went on with increasing drama culminating in a detailed description of the current attack of pain which was so bad that McGlinty could hardly walk. He was living, he claimed, at the house of a friend close to Handlebridge, but was sure he needed to be admitted to hospital in case another operation was necessary and before that, as the pain was so bad, he wanted an injection.

It all sounded highly dubious. Clinical examination showed scars in the right loin, under the right and left costal margins, in the upper abdomen and a large ugly looking one in the right groin. There was slight tenderness on deep pressure just above the umbilicus, but no other signs of disease. The scars certainly corresponded to McGlinty's surgical history, but apart from that his tale was unbelievable. The emergency radiographer was in the hospital and took a plain film of McGlinty's abdomen. Matthew couldn't see much amiss with the pictures, but he called in Peter Allan, the surgical registrar on duty who went through the story again – which was told almost without variation from the first time. The older doctor became quite excited and took Matthew into another room to discuss what he thought.

'Have you ever heard of Munchausen's Syndrome?' he asked. Matthew had, but had never seen a case. 'This is about the most obvious example I have ever seen. Baron von Munchausen was a notorious sixteenth century traveller who told a lot of unlikely stories about his exploits. Richard Asher, who was a physician at the Central Middlesex Hospital, described the condition first and christened it with the Baron's name. Go and look it up in the library when you have a chance. His X-ray does show rather a lot of calcification around the aorta, but there's nothing else to write home about'.

They went back to talk to McGlinty again. 'Is there anywhere we can find out anything about your operations?' asked Allan. 'Do you have a GP?' 'Yes doctor, but I've been moving around for a few weeks since I left my wife and I haven't signed on with anyone else yet.' Allan and Matthew exchanged meaningful glances. 'Where did you used to live and who was your GP then?' 'It was Dr Patel of High Green in Birmingham, doctor. My records should be there.' 'Thank you, we'll ring him up', said Allan politely. 'We don't think there's anything seriously wrong with your tummy – possibly a few adhesions as you said yourself from all the work the surgeons have done on you over the years. The X-ray we took is normal for your age as well. It should all settle down and you don't need an injection. Please come back if you're in the area and the pain gets worse or you start to vomit and we'll do a few more investigations.' And with that, McGlinty protesting a little, but cleared of organic disease, was discharged from the casualty department. Just to make sure, Matthew did look up Dr Patel in the Medical

Directory before he finally let McGlinty go. There was nobody of that name in general practice in High Green, Birmingham.

Matthew Forbes had a few minutes to spare before his casualty shift the following day so he visited the library in the hospital postgraduate centre. He found Richard Asher's famous book *Talking Sense* and turned to the chapter on Munchausen's Syndrome. It made fascinating reading. Laparotomophilia migrans – a wandering lover of laparotomy operations. What a superb definition, he thought to himself. He learned that these patients often bore a grudge against the medical profession and tried to deceive as many doctors as possible, although the repeated operations to which they were prepared to be submitted caused them a great deal of discomfort. Asher had also described two other forms of the syndrome. In one of these the patient tended to feign fits and in the other dramatic bleeding from any orifice in the body. For the sake of satisfying himself that he had not missed anything, Matthew looked up the article which had appeared in the *Lancet* in 1951. The chapter in the book was a straight reprint of the original. Certainly from Asher's descriptions, Patrick McGlinty was a typical Munchausen and it was a good thing, in Matthew's view, that the surgical registrar had managed to spot the diagnosis so quickly and avoid further surgery.

Yet despite the obvious similarities between Matthew Forbes' curious patient in casualty and the cases Richard Asher had described in his book, the young SHO had some doubts. McGlinty had not been resentful in any way except for his comments about the appendectomy which went wrong in adolescence. His various scars fitted in well with his story, however bizarre that might have been. He seemed to be so genuine, except for his name and the unbelieveable events of his florid medical history. Matthew shrugged it off as doctors do when they have other patients and problems to worry about. There could be organic features in McGlinty's story. After all, Asher himself had written 'just as the patient's story is not wholly false, so neither are all the symptoms.' But if Peter Allan, who was his senior, had decided that there was nothing to be done, who was he to disagree? He thought nothing more of his encounter on the previous Monday until three days later when he saw a report from the radiologist about the straight X-ray of McGlinty's abdomen that he had had taken before calling in the registrar. It read as follows:

The only abnormality seen is an excessive degree of calcification in the region just below the origin of the renal vessels. There could be an aneurysm present. Suggest recalling this patient for ultrasound examination.

An *aneurysm*, thought Matthew. That could explain the pain going through to the back if it's beginning to leak. 'Can someone get this man's casualty card out please?', he asked the casualty staff nurse. A few moments later it was on his desk. The address McGlinty had given was ostensibly that of a 'friend' living near Handlebridge. In fact, the house at which he had said he was staying was in Castles Ambo, the neighbouring village to Yewbank where Bill Adams worked, which got its curious name from the fact that it contained two Norman keeps, ambo being ancient English (and incidentally modern Portuguese) for 'both'. The house was called Barbican Cottage, but the casualty clerk had omitted to put the name of the owner of the house on McGlinty's card and there was no telephone number. What to do? Matthew tried to ring the sub-post office in Castles Ambo. Surely they would know the name of the man who lived there if indeed the address was genuine. There was no reply. It was Thursday afternoon – early closing.

Matthew wondered how urgent the problem was. He asked Peter Allan to look at the films and suggest a suitable course of action.

'I doubt whether there's anything seriously wrong here,' said the registrar. 'You remember I commented on the calcification when we saw the film last Monday. That man was as phoney as they come. I'm sure there's no need to do anything quickly.' Then, as if unsure himself, he added 'But you could try ringing the village post office again tomorrow,'

'If the address is genuine after all our trouble,' said Matthew. And then he had another idea. 'I could also ask Dr Adams who works nearby to call in and leave a message while he's on his afternoon round. He carries a car radio and I've got the number in my diary.'

'You do that if you don't think he'll be mad at doing your errands,' threw the registrar over his shoulder as he hurried out of the room looking at his watch. 'Good Lord, is that the time! I'm late for my list already.'

There was no problem at all with contacting Bill Adams on his car radio. 'Castles Ambo', he said, 'yes, we've several patients there. What's the address?' 'Barbican Cottage.' 'Oh that's easy. Old Bert Hodges lives there – has done for years. I don't think he's on the 'phone, but I'll drop a message in to him about his visitor if you like. If your radiologist really thinks that chap has a leaking aneurysm, the sooner you find him the better. Shall I just tell Hodges to get in touch with you at Handle-bridge Hospital and let you know where his friend is now?'

Bill Adams called in at casualty a short while later with some blood samples for the pathology department. 'Hodges wasn't in,' he said, 'I'm sorry I can't help, but I left a note there. He may be away. I know he goes off to visit his son and daughter-in-law quite often. It may be some time before you hear any-thing. Tell me a bit more about your Munchausen. I've never seen one.' And Matthew went over the whole story, which sounded even more unlikely as he told it again to this trainer.

'The trouble is', said the casualty officer unhappily, 'there's no way to find out whether McGlinty is his real name and whether he has a GP.' 'You did ask him the name of his GP, Matthew?' 'Yes, of course. He said it was a Dr Patel of High Green, a suburb of Birmingham. I've looked him up in the Medical Directory and there's no GP by that name working in High Green, as far as I can tell.' 'You keep a medical directory in casualty?' 'Yes, Bill. They let us have the old ones from the Postgraduate Library as soon as they get their new edition.' 'What date is the one you used?' 'Oh, I don't know. Let's have a look . . . It's 1985.' 'Three years out of date, so it doesn't mean a thing. Why don't you either look up Dr Patel in a current medical register or ring the Birmingham Family Practitioner Committee and ask them if they have a doctor of that name working in High Green?' 'I can't get hold of a medical register at the moment, but I'll have a word with the switchboard and ask them to ring Birmingham' said Matthew, and did just that.

A short while later he was on the 'phone to the Birmingham

FPC. 'There *is* a Dr Patel working in High Green you say? Dr Harish Patel. Do you have his number? Thank you.' He turned to Bill Adams, his face alight with a new enthusiasm. 'This should be interesting,' he said. 'I think we're about to learn something important.'

It was about four in the afternoon and Matthew was not too hopeful about contacting Dr Patel at his surgery, but to his surprise he got through at once. 'Yes, this is Dr Patel speaking.' A soft clear Indian voice. 'Patrick McGlinty, you say. Yes, I know him well. Funny name he has for a Cockney, but I think his father was Irish and they settled in the East End of London. I did my vocational training there after leaving Guy's and we've chatted about the area when he's been to see me. I saw his wife last week and she told me they'd had a row some time ago and they've split up. Not surprising after all the times he's been off round the world on exploring trips leaving her at home. You may have read about the last expedition he went on about five years ago. That man with the funny name Smite . . . something was returning to do some work in the Congo and took McGlinty with him because he's so experienced in tropical travel. He had to be flown back home in an emergency. Just a minute, I'll get his notes out.' There was a brief pause. 'It's a very thick file, but he's had a lot of trouble. Ah yes, if I remember correctly, the main problem he's had is that nobody believes him when he tells them the story of his exploits. There's one letter in here from Bristol which said he was thought to have Munchausen's Syndrome and they're not the only ones who have got it wrong. All his abdominal troubles are absolutely genuine.' Matthew exchanged a few more pleasantries with the helpful Dr Patel and then rang off.

'How wrong can you be?' he said to his trainer, with some concern. 'Now what do we do?' 'You've certainly got a problem' said the GP. 'He could be anywhere in Britain. Your only hope is that he's still staying with Bert Hodges and that he'll get in touch soon. You could put out an emergency call through the police or local radio either for Hodges or for McGlinty himself to ring you. Anyway – good luck! I must get back for evening surgery. Tell me how you get on.'

Medicine is a curious business. Sometimes things go dreadfully wrong. Patients get fobbed off with the wrong diagnosis and go and die totally avoidable deaths following which everybody turns on the unfortunate physician whose reputation up till then may have been impeccable. As Mark Antony said 'the evil that men do lives after them. The good is oft interred with their bones.' Thoughts something like these were whirling round in Matthew Forbes' head as, sitting with his hands round a cup of tea in the casualty office, he pondered what to do about his mistaken Munchausen. The worst fear of all was of McGlinty keeling over suddenly in the street, his abdomen filling up with blood cascading out of his ruptured aortic aneursym. His reverie was brought to an abrupt halt by the male charge nurse in the doorway.

'Sorry to disturb you, Matthew,' he said. 'But I think we've got our Munchausen back again. He's telling an even odder story now about you asking to see him.' The need to preserve a macho image usually prevents young SHOs from throwing their arms round members of the same sex. But Matthew nearly did.

'Send him in, send him in,' he beamed at the startled charge nurse who was not expecting a reaction like this. 'So you got our message, Mr McGlinty. Thank you for coming back, is the pain still bad?' It was, but it was no worse and there was no mass to feel in McGlinty's battle-scarred abdomen.

The rest is all good news. The radiologist carried out an ultrasound scan, which confirmed an aortic aneurysm which was probably beginning to leak. The vascular surgeon, assisted by Peter Allan, who was far too good a doctor to be upset for long by his wrong diagnosis, soon cut out the diseased aorta and put in a graft. McGlinty recovered well from the operation and made it up with his wife, who came down to Castles Ambo to stay with Bert Hodges until the pair of them could go back to Birmingham. And Matthew Forbes? He went through his vocational training with flying colours and joined Bill Adams as a partner soon afterwards. But he never forgot about Munchausen's Syndrome. 'Most cases resemble organic emergencies,' wrote Richard Asher. One of them, Matthew reflected frequently, nearly was.

JOHN WOODWARD
Sidcup

Freud described the two great motives in life: aggression and sex. A third could be added: the desire for publicity.

The Test

At the age of fifty Hector was driven by a desperate wish to avoid medical anonymity. He saw himself not so much an unfledged Cromwell – a surgeon can hardly plead that he is 'guiltless of his countrie's blood' – but rather a mute inglorious Lister. It was so unfair. In other, more prestigious hospitals, colleagues never let an operating session pass without separating Siamese triplets or transplanting at least one heart. His own days in theatre were mundane catalogues of bread-and-butter surgery – varicose veins, hernias, piles and breast lumps. Useful toil, no doubt, but he felt distinctly 'mocked by ambition' whenever he tried to persuade some supercilious teaching hospital registrar to accept the transfer of one of his more difficult cases.

He looked despairingly again at the envelope which represented yet another setback in his efforts to achieve clinical apotheosis. It contained what a writer would call a 'rejection slip', although since it was from a medical journal it took the form of a lengthy letter from the editor accompanied by referees' reports. The net effect was still the same. His increasingly dog-eared manuscript had once more done its imitation of a pigeon with end-stage homesickness.

Edmond Hector had a buccal bee in his bonnet. As the alimentary tract is continuous he felt that anything happening in one part of it must be reflected throughout its length. He had therefore taken to examining smears from the mouths of all his patients to search for signs in which he contrived to see potential bowel cancer years before it could otherwise be expected to manifest itself. The longer he pursued his theory, the more numerous and more subtle became the stages of pre-disease that he categorised.

When this latter-day haruspex* found, as he frequently did,

*In ancient Rome, a diviner or soothsayer who foretold the fortune by the inspection of the entrails of animals (Ed.).

the stigmata he sought, he advocated preventive measures in keeping with the alternative spirit of the day. These consisted predominantly of meditation and the prescription of somewhat unpalatable diets. Certain foods were arbitrarily deemed carcinogenic. When a repeat smear was taken after six months of thought and dieting Hector invariably saw a vast improvement in the buccal smear.

He was finding it hard to persuade other doctors of the significance of his results. He had been philosophical about being spurned by the *British Medical Journal* and the *Lancet*, publications to which he and other members of the British Stomach and Bowel Society referred dismissively as 'The Weekly Comics'. However, this latest rejection was from *Belly*, the Society's own esoteric and esteemed journal. He felt very hurt.

He knew that the work was valid. The trouble was that it was ahead of its time. He had done for bowel cancer what Papanicolaou had done for cancer of the cervix. In a little flight of fancy he saw the name of Hector taking its place alongside those of Graves, Hodgkin, Addison – Hippocrates even. He would be joining that élite group whose identities are indissolubly linked with a disease or a clinical sign, an eponymous custom nowadays rather frowned on by the orthodox, who feel that 'Fabry's Disease' is somehow less memorable, and less indicative, of the underlying disease process than 'angiokeratoma corporis diffusum'. Sour grapes perhaps?

He read the paper through again. If he could only get it published it would boost both himself and his hospital in the eyes of his peers. There must be something else he could do. The time had come to cut a few corners. He thought briefly, then lifted the phone. Perhaps he could relieve some of the pain of this latest rejection by enlisting the analgesic pencil of a local journalist whose appendix he had removed a few month's previously. The resulting paragraph was short but satisfactory. If anything Hector was a little staggered by how emphatic it was. He had not allowed for the journalistic tendency to ignore the qualifying remarks with which scientists and doctors (the two groups being otherwise almost completely incongruent) hedge everything they say.

'Thousands of lives could be saved by a test pioneered at

Granton General Hospital by one of the country's top surgeons. In an exclusive interview with *The Advertiser* he said that the test – which takes tissue from inside the cheek and can detect stomach and bowel cancer before it develops – is cheap and simple to carry out. The results are soon to be published in a leading medical journal'.

He liked the 'top surgeon' bit but wished that a 'leading medical journal' actually was about to publish his article. Perhaps this would put a little pressure on one of them; they could hardly ignore him now. Had Edmond Hector been a limited company with a Stock Exchange quotation there was enough in that paragraph to raise the value of his shares by fifty pence or more overnight – as happens to drug firms which announce a 'possible cure for AIDS' on the strength of some tenuous observation in a couple of mice.

If Hector had expected his phone call to the local paper to be a one-day wonder he had badly miscalculated. Cancer ranks second only to the sexual indiscretions of the minor clergy in the appetite of the media-consuming public. Add to that the vogue for interpreting 'preventive medicine' as being synonymous with the conferring of immortality, a modern *Elixir Vitae*, and the scope was there for organs more influential than *The Advertiser* to grab. And grab they did, not hesitating in the process to disparage the blinkered vision of a medical profession which was yet again slow to take up a new development which was not hi-tech enough to feed its self-esteem.

Hector didn't have to be asked twice to appear on television. Only after he had accepted did any doubt creep in. It might have been better to wait until the article had been published before launching out quite so publicly. He knew it was simply a matter of time before everyone shared his opinion about the value of the test but he promised himself that he would not make excessively rash claims during the interview. In the event, of course, what he said was largely determined by factors outside his control.

'How many lives will this test save, doctor?' the presenter began.

Hector ignored the honorary title so irritating to surgeons

who, for reasons best known to themselves, like to retain their links with the barber-shops of the last century.

'Sixteen thousand people die of bowel cancer in this country every year; another five thousand from stomach cancer. That is ten times the incidence of cancer of the neck of the womb – yet we have a vast screening programme for that fairly rare disease. Of course it is a feminist issue and politically sensitive so it attracts interest – and funds – out of all proportion to its importance.'

'Is this the first test of its kind?'

'There is a much less accurate one based on looking at samples of – er – solid excreta. It has never been possible to persuade people to take that up on any large scale. You can see why. In any case it only finds established disease. My test is quite straightforward. Anyone will be able to take it from themselves, made a slide and send it to their nearest hospital.'

'What proof do you have that your diets work? After all, no one seems really sure that cervical screening prevents many deaths.' The presenter had obviously been briefed by the studio's medical adviser.

'The changes are readily seen in the repeat smears. It is perfectly obvious that if you treat a pre-cancerous lesion and it disappears then the method has worked,' replied Hector. 'We can't afford to sit around waiting for evidence on morbidity and mortality which will take years to collect. Scepticism must not stand in the way of progress.'

'I am not sure how you know whether something is precancerous if you don't see it change into cancer. However, what you seem to be saying is that no one need ever again die from bowel cancer?' concluded the presenter.

'That is putting things a bit strongly, but certainly the incidence should be greatly reduced.'

Since most people – even other journalists – only attend to any programme with half an ear, it was not surprising that the echoes of the interview in various broadcasts and in magazines and papers later either attributed to Hector the remark 'No-one need ever die of bowel cancer again', or alternatively blazed 'Cancer Doc slates greedy women'.

In a few short minutes Hector had upset not only the medical establishment but also a large proportion of the female population of Britain. Nevertheless, his test grasped the public imagination. The notion that bowel cancer could be prevented by simply taking a smear from the mouth had immediate popular appeal. The average patient has as much enthusiasm for being invaded by a doctor as the average feminist has for being invaded by a male.

The Trade Union Congress passed a motion emphasising the right of every working man and woman to have a buccal smear. Hector received correspondence by the sackful from people demanding the test. There were letters by MPs from the Scillies to the Shetlands insisting that he add one or more of their constituents to his waiting list immediately. These trans-border referrals were naturally in full accordance with DHSS policy that the public should shop round all the hospitals in the National Health Service to find the one they liked best.

To his surprise he also received quite a lot of support from a number of medical colleagues, some of whom even began to out-Herod Herod. There were soon parts of the country in which family doctors knew that the merest hint of an intestinal problem in a referral letter was a guarantee of an instant out-patient appointment. In those same areas anyone with Irrita-ble Bowel Syndrome entering the wards would be endos-coped, Cat-scanned and, of course, buccally smeared, within a couple of hours of admission. Matters less fashionable and less fascinating – the ruptured aortae, the cardiac arrests, the diabetic comas – were not accorded quite the same degree of urgency. When the interest of a consultant and the interests of a community fail to coincide, the consultant generally prevails.

Consequently, Hector had some answers when challenged a few months later in a further television interview by a predict-ably reactionary London Professor who claimed to be unable to replicate his results.

'You have not copied my methods precisely. It is an ex-tremely sensitive test and it has to be done exactly as I have described. It is comment enough to say that many other hospi-tals, such as those in Bettws-y-Coed and St Bees, are getting results comparable with mine.'

'And the Emperor had new clothes. We are not talking about

cooking – where two people can follow the same recipe and end up with dishes which are totally different,' shouted the Professor. 'In science anyone following the same procedures should get the same answer. There is no such thing as scientific "Green Fingers", you know.'

'I'm afraid you have a bad case of the NIH syndrome,' snapped Hector. 'NIH? What is that?' intervened the presenter. 'Not Invented Here. It is usually a rather chauvinist sort of argument – you know, "Not British", so "No good". This time it is just because a small out-of-the-way district hospital has shown that it can teach the big boys a thing or two. The good Professor seems to expect *Ex Granton nunquam aliquid novi*, if I may adapt Pliny.'

'Granton is a trifle less exotic and considerably less varied than Africa. May I remind you that Pliny also wrote *Ne supra crepideam sutor iudicaret*.'

'I don't think all our viewers will quite have your grasp of Greek. Could you explain, please,' purred the interviewer. 'Roughly – the cobbler should stick to his last. I am sure that Mr Hector is an excellent district hospital surgeon – a general practitioner of provincial surgery, if you like. I could not do his job properly and he cannot do mine – complex research is a field for the professionals.'

The outraged Hector had to be forcibly restrained by the studio crew.

His colleagues in his own hospital were half proud of the recognition, half irritated by the effect of Hector's repeated absences on their own workload. Even when he was not lecturing or fund-raising he was too busy with the smears to do such trivial things as participating in the 'on-call' rota.

As word about the test filtered down into the lower reaches of the medical columns of women's magazines and into pamphlets on the walls of citizens advice bureaux, Hector began to find himself beseiged by patients who wanted the test, however irrelevant to their condition – though he himself found it hard to imagine circumstances in which it could ever be totally irrelevant. To be fair to him, he had shown remarkable self-restraint for a surgeon; the only treatment he ever recommended on the strength of his test was dietary.

Although there had been stories from other countries of Hectorean disciples who had, as it were, taken his teaching to its logical conclusion, he was rather startled to find a young woman in his clinic one day who was prepared to press him to go beyond his culinary prestidigitation. He had told her that she had a positive smear test. She demanded surgery.

'It is my right to have it. I cannot live for six months wondering whether the diet is going to work. I insist that you do something. I'll even pay you if I must.'

Pretty young women presumably often choose their operations à la carte in streets where faces are commercially elevated and bosoms refashioned for a consideration. Edmond Hector's singularly unmercantile experience had failed to teach him how to explain diplomatically that prophylactic colectomies were not included in the surgical menu he offered. Nevertheless, despite considerable pressure from the girl he resisted. He had never been quite certain of the meaning of the expression 'in high dudgeon' but rather suspected that her manner on leaving the clinic epitomised it.

It was evening once again. The glimmering landscape of Granton General Hospital faded on the sight. A solemn silence held the air in Edmond Hector's office. He had reached the end of a busy day scraping the cheeks of half the county and was belatedly opening the mail which still avalanched daily into the room. Suddenly he stopped. Two envelopes, one brown, one expensively white, held letters very different from the routine smear requests. When he had read them both he sat back in disbelief.

The brown envelope contained an invitation from the General Medical Council to account for his television interview. Apart from the deadly sin of advertising his own skills, he had made claims about his test which were not supported by published data and specifically had stated that no one need die of bowel cancer. In short, he was accused of being a publicity seeking fraud.

In the white envelope was a letter from the solicitor of the young woman to whom he had denied the prophylactic colectomy. It alleged negligence in that he had not provided all necessary treatment, so compelling her to find another surgeon to give her, at considerable expense, what she wanted. She was looking for financial compensation both for the inconvenience and for the mental stress occasioned by having to wait for surgery while knowing that she carried cells within her that might explode into malignancy at any moment. The solicitor reserved the right to have a second bite at the cherry at any time in the lifetime of his client – or indeed later still – should the delay prove to have permitted the spread of microscopic disease.

It was a fork Morton himself would have been proud to devise. It was a fork to turn Karpov's bilberry yoghurt green with envy. He could only defend himself against the one charge by effectively pleading guilty to the other. It looked as if he was going to get his wish. He would not die 'to fortune and to fame unknown'. The name of Hector would be recorded in the annals of medicine, though hardly in a way he had envisaged. Edmond Hector made a mental note. In one respect Thomas Gray had got it wrong.

The Paths of Glory lead but to the Courts.

ROBERT ROUSE
Colwyn Bay

8
Doctor–Patient Relationships: Awkward Patients

Plato, in 410 BC, when advising about healthy living, condemned the 'excessive care for the body that goes beyond simple gymnastics . . . for the person is forever imagining headaches and dizziness . . . It makes the man always fancy himself sick and never cease from anguishing about his body.'[11] And Karl Marx, the distinguished medical scholar, stated that 'Physicians see many "diseases" which have no more real existence than an image in the mirror'.[12] Indeed the hypochondriac with multiple symptoms provides a problem for every doctor. It is difficult to alter the patient's persistent belief in non-existent illness and his or her fear and preoccupation with disease. The doctor, while giving the essential reassurance, is always worried about missing the development of organic disease.

An example of a male hypochondriac who had an unfortunate accident follows:

The Troubles of Rotarian Church

In the twenty years since he had been a patient on Dr David Scott's list, Benjamin Church had called in the doctor or attended the health centre in the main square of Trillington on no fewer than four hundred and thirty-five occasions, making an average of nearly twenty-two times a year. In fact, the partners in the group practice had started a sweepstake on when he would reach the notable milestone of five hundred consultations, an event not difficult to predict as his requests for medical assistance were a remarkably regular occurrence. Church was an ironmonger in his early fifties. He was also a hypochondriac. Whatever else might be said of him, of this, as W.S. Gilbert once said about something else, there was 'no possible, probable manner of doubt.'

Mr Church was also a Rotarian, not that this had anything to do with his valetudinarian tendencies, for the club is a worthy and dignified institution and does much good in the community. Benjamin's wife Connie, a gentle and uncomplaining soul, had put up with Benjamin's obvious enjoyment of chronic ill health for the whole of their marriage. There were no children, which was a pity because the young are forthright in their opinions and would have told their pathetic father in no uncertain terms to stop being a waste of space and get on with living. Connie had always hankered after a pet as a child-substitute, but the choice was somewhat limited. Dogs were forbidden in the home because Benjamin had read about *Toxocara canis*, that notorious parasitic worm of the dog intestine which, when spread to man, can infect the human retina. Benjamin was sure he would go blind if he had so much as patted one. Nor were cats any better for he had heard dreadful tales about the transmission of toxoplasmosis, which is an organism of one cell like the amoeba, carried by cats and transmitted to man in whom it can infect the brain, although this is rare in adults who are healthy. Eventually, after much hard work by Connie, who had roped in Dr Scott for support, Benjamin was persuaded that the risk of psittacosis or parrot fever was minimal and a budgerigar was admitted to the household.

The bird Connie chose was a blue male, decidedly surly in behaviour and inclined to sit morosely in a corner of his cage resisting all attempts to induce him to say 'pretty boy' or 'hallo'. Christened Nelson, because Benjamin was a great admirer of Britain's most famous sea-dog, the miserable creature remained grammatically mute for three years, although he squawked out a few unintelligible expletives whenever a finger was offered to him as a friendly gesture. Then the great day arrived when he said his first words. With a perfect expression of intense suffering, learned by many months of perceptive modelling, he put his head on his wing, half closed his eyes and piped mournfully in a high-pitched whine exactly like Benjamin in one of his crises 'Call the doctor, dear.'

It is not that Benjamin was an unpleasant person. His friends knew him as a charming and generous companion, provided one was not foolish enough to broach the subject of health, and most of them were sufficiently experienced to avoid that pitfall. The family business of Wilfrid Church and Son, started by his grandfather in 1910, had an excellent name for reliability and Benjamin had retained many grateful customers despite the opening of a do-it-yourself supermarket on Trillington's busy by-pass. He regularly stood out in the town square in the bitterest of weather collecting for the Rotary Club in aid of one charity or another and his abode was an open house to anybody who chose to call. But of all the guests in his home, it was the doctor whom he welcomed with the most widely open arms and as often as possible, because unlike his fellow Rotarians and other acquaintances, the hapless fellow was under contract to listen to Benjamin's morbid obsession with each aspect of his bodily functions.

Benjamin Church had read everything he could about medical matters. He did not waste time with *The Home Doctor*, but at enormous expense bought each twin volume edition of the *Oxford Textbook of Medicine* as soon as it was published and scanned its detailed pages avidly for new knowledge as often as he could. He knew the symptoms of angina pectoris, diverticulitis, cancer of every part of the body and all the collagen diseases, especially the rare ones. His most notable skill was the recognition of the earliest signs of skin disorders on his own cuticle and he believed that every miniscule blemish should be made to vanish immediately with hydrocortisone as soon as he had shared its presence with his despairing doctor.

The arrival of myalgic encephalomyelitis (ME to its friends) on the medical scene was like manna from heaven for Benjamin. This long-lasting state of debility, which is thought to follow a virus infection and is especially common after glandular fever, has no diagnostic tests and so cannot be proved or disproved to be present by clinical science. The diagnosis is subjective and although no doubt many cases are genuine, it also attracts several professional patients each year to a foothold on its bandwagon. With ME, Benjamin had, at last, an irrefutable answer for his lethargy and his aches and pains, a clear sign that his neurasthenic problems were rooted not in his 'nerves' as his doctor was always saying, but in established physical disease. He became an actively contributing member of the ME Society, donating vast sums for the propagation of the association's aims and objectives and rapidly wore into silence every officer in that highly articulate organisation with the incessant chronicling of his protean symptoms.

It was not surprising that over the years each of the other partners in Trillington Health Centre came to know Benjamin Church very well. Deputising for David Scott while he was given a temporary respite made contact with the neurotic ironmonger almost inevitable. The other doctors could hardly be blamed for their ribaldry on the frequent occasions that his name was mentioned, for it was the only way to remain sane while responding to his outrageous demands.

Trillington Rotary Club always held its annual ladies' night at the Croaking Frog. Dignitaries from brother clubs were invited as honoured guests and chief among them was the Area President, who during his year in office could live very comfortably on fodder provided entirely by his official engagements. There was a suitably grand ballroom on the first floor of the hostelry and it was traditional to stage a sit-down dinner with toasts and speeches followed by a dance. This year, however, the year that Benjamin was to experience real illness for the very first time in his life, was to be different.

For a variety of reasons, the club's social committee had decided at its organising meeting to scale down ladies' night. One of the factors involved was the cost which had risen out of all proportion to the quality of the food. But the main cause of the change of plan was that the previous year's banquet had been an unmitigated disaster. The Trillington President had found a cockroach in his soup and his honoured guest, the Chairman of another men's club in the town called the Profound Table, as well as his lady and half a dozen others had developed acute staphylococcal poisoning from the sorbet which came on with dramatic effect during the last waltz. The manager of the Croaking Frog was full of apologies and promised it would never happen again, but these were not isolated incidents, as other diners-out had also noticed a general deterioration in the cuisine. There was no other suitable venue in the town for the most important function on the Trillington Rotary Calendar. So this year would be a compromise. The club would use the ballroom in the Croaking Frog, but only on condition that it could have a buffet prepared by an outside caterer. The guests would be invited to collect their canapés, quiches lorraine, sausages on sticks and other delicacies and seat themselves at tables round the dance floor.

Benjamin and Connie arrived in good time and joined fellow Rotarians and their wives at the bar. The evening progressed smoothly with the usual convivial atmosphere of Trillington Ladies' Night, and the buffet was rapidly divided onto two hundred groaning plates on the ballroom tables. The Area President, Giles Cattermole-Jones, the guest of honour, came from Castlehurst, a town about thirty miles away from Trillington and Benjamin had never met him, but his wife looked vaguely familiar. She was a woman of about his own age he thought, heavily made up and decked out in a brilliant and very expensive red gown. It was the epitomy of what Oliver Goldsmith once called 'the glaring impotence of dress'. She and her husband passed close by the Church's table. For a brief second her eyes met Benjamin's and that look was his undoing, for in a flash he recognised her. It was a pity that his mouth was full, because its contents, with the exception of his false teeth, went at least part of the way down the wrong tube. He spluttered, turned blue, began to lose consciousness and was only saved by Paul Blake, an astute companion on his table who just happened to be the chief surgeon at Trillington Royal Infirmary. Blake carried out a successful Heimlich manoeuvre which propelled the obstruction back into Benjamin's mouth whereon he gratefully swallowed it down the correct passage. Understandably shaken, Benjamin was taken home in a taxi after he had regained some composure and except for some discomfort in his epigastrium (Paul Blake was a powerful man) he appeared the following morning to be little the worse for his frightening experience.

So what was it about Mrs Cattermole-Jones which so nearly led to Benjamin's early demise? Here I must be discreet, for the details never were completely known. Suffice it to say that twenty years previously, when Benjamin was not much more than thirty, Connie had been called away to look after her ailing mother in Newcastle, leaving Benjamin to fend for himself for a month. Old Wilfrid would not hear of his grandson deserting his duties in the shop. One day a local girl called Gloria Virago, flashily attractive, twice-divorced and quite ruthless had appeared in the ironmonger's and chatted him up. Things progressed and before Connie's return the single-minded young woman had managed to visit Benjamin's flat, and the rest I leave to your imagination.

Benjamin had never told Connie about it. It remained the one much-dreaded skeleton in his cupboard. You may have thought that Gloria would have tried to compete when the troubles with Connie's mother were over, but by then she had realised that Benjamin, though an excellent ironmonger, knew very little about the mysteries of passionate love and had cast her lascivious eyes elsewhere. Cattermole-Jones had proved a much better proposition and had whisked her away out of Benjamin's acutely embarrassed life until their fateful reunion at the Croaking Frog.

Reader, it would be nice to end the story there with Benjamin's secret intact and his café choking effectively treated, but you know that life is not like that. Over the next few days, he developed discomfort in the upper part of his abdomen and Connie rang Dr Scott.

'How bad is it, Connie?' he said, obviously unwilling to be committed to yet another visit to the Church household.

'Well, David, I know he does go on a bit about his health, but he had this nasty shock last Saturday night – I expect Paul told you about it – and he wonders whether he has a broken rib.'

'Can't he come down to the Health Centre?'

'It would be difficult, as he can't manage the car because of the pain and you know I can't drive.'

'It would be quicker if he did come here. I might not be able to see him until after evening surgery if I have to make a call.'

David went through all the tricks of a family doctor who feels himself getting cornered by a persistent patient. Who could blame him? This incident in Benjamin's life was to prove the first genuine serious physical illness in his medical history and it was very nearly his last, but at this stage David Scott was not to know that. To his ears it sounded like one more futile episode in Benjamin's relentless progression towards his five-hundredth consultation.

Eventually, Scott decided that he would waste as much time by wriggling on the end of the 'phone as dragging himself round to the Church's home. Benjamin certainly did not look very well. He bore a subdued expression, unusual for him as he was generally animated in presenting his symptoms. There was little to glean from going further into the history. He had, as Connie had said, a great deal of residual tenderness below each costal margin where Paul Blake's enormous hands had pumped his dinner out of his larynx, but no evidence that his spleen or liver had been damaged and few definite signs of a fractured rib. His temperature was normal and David Scott found nothing in his chest to suggest pneumonia, which he certainly looked for in view of the fact that Benjamin could easily have inhaled a particle of food into his lungs. It seemed that the most likely diagnosis to explain the vague abdominal discomfort was a viral gastritis, and Scott asked Connie to go and get Benjamin a bottle of magnesium trisilicate. He left with the invitation to them to get in touch if the trouble did not settle down in a few days.

It didn't. Connie was on the 'phone again three days later to say that Benjamin was worse. When Scott called he saw at once that she was right. The patient looked extremely unwell. He was sweating slightly and had a temperature of 101 (Scott never could use the Centigrade Scale). His chest remained clear, but although Blake's bruising had settled down there was now definite tenderness over the stomach. Despite this, Benjamin had normal bowel actions and had not vomited although his appetite was reduced to virtually nothing. Scott checked a mid-stream urine which was normal and carried out a full blood count and ESR. The latter was quite high at forty-six, and Benjamin's white cell count showed an increase in neutrophils – findings which suggested infection somewhere. By this time Scott was getting slightly worried. His colleagues, however, were highly amused when Benjamin's case was discussed over coffee and few of them thought that there would be a serious organic cause for his troubles. Crying 'wolf' is the most dangerous game a patient can play.

When Benjamin showed no signs of improvement after a week, David Scott rang the Royal Infirmary and spoke to Paul Blake. 'It doesn't really sound a surgical problem, David,' Blake said. 'I think it would be a good idea to let the physicians work on him first and I'll see him if they get stuck.'

Scott then contacted John England, the gastroenterologist, who agreed to admit Benjamin the same day for investigation. A short while later, his registrar Carol King rang the Trillington practice with some results.

'We think it's sub-acute bacterial endocarditis,' she said. 'His ESR has gone up to sixty-eight and we've grown a *strep.* from his blood culture. His spleen's enlarged as well and there's a definite systolic murmur. We've started him on large doses of penicillin by injection and already he's a bit better. He should be able to come home in a few days.'

Benjamin did come home a short while later, now on oral penicillin, and seemed to be getting over his infection. Of course, he looked up endocarditis in his voluminous textbook and was a trifle startled by what he read. David Scott had to pour large volumes of oil on decidedly troubled waters during his frequent post-discharge visits. A week after leaving hospital however, his condition suddenly took a turn for the worse. It happened on a Sunday morning when Scott's trainee, Malcolm Davis, was on duty. Benjamin was smitten with acute abdominal pain in the small hours which started in the area of his umbilicus. He vomited, had a single loose motion and noticed that the pain then moved to being low down in the right side.

Malcolm was a straightforward young man who favoured a no-nonsense approach. 'You've got appendicitis, Mr Church,' he said cheerfully. 'I don't know how it all ties up with your other problems, but there's no doubt about it and I'll send you back into hospital at once.' There was some difficulty with Paul Blake's house surgeon, who whinged about not having any beds, but Malcolm Davis had been through the vocational training scheme for general practice at the Infirmary and soon managed to negotiate that obstacle with a few well-chosen words like 'Didn't I hear Blake say once that acute cases were to be admitted without any questions from the Trillington Practice – to the gynae ward if necessary?' and more devastating still 'Weren't you the chap who was talking in the postgraduate centre the other day about wanting to apply for the GP training scheme after your pre-reg. jobs?'

Benjamin was duly admitted and the signs Malcolm had described were confirmed by the surgical registrar. A fairly urgent operation seemed to be the only course of action. Before the eager young doctors could plunge their knives into him, Benjamin made a request to be allowed to be treated privately. 'Mr Blake is a personal friend and a fellow-Rotarian,' he pleaded. 'If I'm going to die I'd rather he saw me first.' And with that he sank back onto his plastic casualty pillow and re-signed himself to his fate. Paul Blake came in, of course, and had a look at him, but realising that to take him on as a private patient would mean that he would never be able to escape from Benjamin's hypochondriasis, he elected to look after him on the NHS. Blake contacted John England, who was having a round of golf before his Sunday dinner, and after weighing up the pros and cons together it was decided to operate without delay.

'We'll do a laparotomy,' said Blake to his house surgeon who was assisting him. 'That's because it isn't quite typical of an appendix and so I'll make an incision nearer to the mid-line in case we have to have a wider look round. Do you know how laparotomy got its name?' The house surgeon didn't, or chose not to say so if he did, because he knew how Blake liked to show off to the theatre sister. 'No classical scholars left in medicine now, sister,' he grumbled. 'It's from the Greek word *laparos* meaning "soft" and stands for any incision into the soft abdomen – get it?' The house surgeon nodded glumly and stood ready with a pair of artery forceps to clamp off bleeding vessels after Blake's scalpel had left a scarlet gorge in Benjamin's abdomen.

I expect, reader, with your clinical acumen, you have already diagnosed the trouble and know full well what Blake found when he probed inside the unfortunate ironmonger's tummy. The obvious is often farthest from the mind. Perhaps a more careful history would have spotted the cause earlier; after all it *did* start immediately after Ladies' Night and of all the clinicians who had been involved in Benjamin's care, Paul Blake should have been the one to have remembered what happened at his table. Anyway, even if he had forgotten, it all came back to him like the light on Damascus Road when, with a startled gasp and then a gesture of triumph he removed the plastic cocktail stick that had perforated Benjamin's caecum.

There is little more to tell. The physicians all had red faces. 'SBE indeed!' hissed Blake whenever he saw one in the corridor. They in their turn made snide comments about Heimlich manoeuvres which forced cocktail sticks into the gullet. The news went round Trillington Rotary like wildfire – it even filtered through to other clubs in the area and Benjamin's convalescence in hospital was nearly destroyed by a get-well card bearing the Castlehurst postmark which contained the message 'I did recognise you at the dinner, Darling. We must meet up again soon.' David Scott won the sweepstake on Benjamin's five-hundredth consultation. He had opted for a date six months earlier than his partners and of course Benjamin's *bona fide* illness inevitably brought that milestone forward. Connie and Benjamin still live more or less happily in Trillington, but Benjamin hasn't changed. He is well on his way to his thousandth doctor contact, but David Scott takes some comfort from the fact that by then he will probably have retired from general practice. Oh, and I nearly forgot. Nelson picked up a new word which he screeched from his cage whenever anybody came into the room. Laparotomy . . .

JOHN WOODWARD
Sidcup

Most patients can be recognised as belonging to certain groups. The well read, argumentative, intelligent person who can easily 'fix' his doctor is always a challenge[13]

Worm's Eye View

It had to be a doctor, of course, who made the observation that 'some women cannot see a telephone without taking the receiver off'. I do not believe that the Headmaster and his wife had ever been patients of Somerset Maugham but, nevertheless the description was particularly appropriate.

At first sight they appeared to be an ill-matched couple. She was large, Amazonian and forbidding. She always brought to mind a description by Stephen Leacock – 'a parallelogram – that is, an oblong angular figure, which cannot be described, but which is equal to anything'. She commanded a fearful respect (or should it be respectful fear?) from all who knew her, and appeared to be the dominant partner in the union.

He, on the other hand, was meek and inoffensive with sleeked-down greying hair and a meticulously straight centre parting. He spent much of his spare time since his retirement alone in his study where he was surrounded by his books, mainly in Latin and Ancient Greek (he had a second in Greats from Oxford). He did, however, have an incongruous interest. He was a self-taught expert on single malt whisky, which liquid he did not, unfortunately, share with me when I had occasion to visit him professionally. I suspect that he consumed a fair quantity of the Highland nectar while reading Horace, or Tacitus, or Plato as a means of escaping the attention of his wife.

They had two children. The son, who was in his mid-twenties, was a post-graduate student at the London School of Economics and he appeared to make economies in such essential commodities as soap and water as, on the rare occasions that he ventured North to visit his parents, he always appeared with the same long greasy coiffure, the same grimy greyness of his facial skin and the same corduroy trousers reminiscent of the operating frock coat of a pre-Lister surgeon, in that they were so encrusted with grease they would probably have remained standing even had the wearer vacated them. He inevitably addressed people as 'comrade'.

The daughter, a few years younger than her brother, was pale and thin with long straight blonde hair and preferred to wear kaftans and thus the overall effect was like a hairy wigwam. She was reading sociology at a 'white tile' university on the south coast. She marched for all the fashionable causes ('Americans out of Vietnam') but not for the unfashionable ones ('Russians out of Czechoslovakia'). She shared a flat with a male soulmate who was training to be a journalist. She, too, avoided the long journey to her parents' home as often as she could.

If the Headmaster and his wife were perturbed by the indifference of their offspring they hid it well, for they always spoke of their children with the most glowing fondness, although their love for them was almost totally unrequited.

This, then, was the background to a family with whom I had had only occasional contacts until my life became inextricably entwined with theirs one Sunday evening in late summer. I was having my evening meal, already delayed because of a visit to an asthmatic child, when my mince (I couldn't afford to pay the mortgage *and* eat beef in those days) and potatoes were disturbed again by the cacophonous jangle of the telephone bell. (Those of you with long memories will be able to recall the days when 'phones rang; nowadays they warble and bleep – and very often fail to waken me!) It was the Headmaster's wife imperiously demanding my presence forthwith, as her spouse had been smitten with severe abdominal pain. I left the meal and drove the four miles across town to the patient's house. It was the end of the Glasgow holidays and the start of the Edinburgh ones (or vice-versa) and traffic was at a standstill as the narrow city-centre streets were choked in both directions. I took forty-five minutes to reach the house to find an extremely agitated wife and a quieter and, by now, partially recovered husband. The pain, which had been peri-umbilical, had largely disappeared and physical signs were absent. I muttered words like 'bowel spasm' and 'inflammation and colic' but I don't think that they believed them any more readily than I did. We reached a bargain; they would telephone me if there was any change in his condition and I would visit him again the following morning.

With a certain sense of foreboding I returned home. My meal had long since passed the point of edibility, so I went to bed hungry and took some time to fall asleep. I was roused by the telephone: it was the Headmaster's wife to tell me that her husband had opened his bowels and was now feeling considerably better. ('You did say to ring if there was any change, doctor'.) I thanked her as profusely as the circumstances would permit and tried to fall asleep: it took over an hour.

Next day, feeling somewhat under par, I revisited as arranged. The patient was lying in bed with his wife standing guard and answering his questions for him: he still had a few niggly pains but was otherwise feeling well. There was, however, an air of apprehension about him. I thought of Balint and asked what I thought were searching and appropriate questions. Eventually I made the breakthrough.

'Is it appendicitis, doctor?' he asked. 'You see, my father died with a perforated appendix.'

I assured him that there were no signs of that and he appeared to relax. He talked about his recent visit to Speyside where he had discovered a single malt unknown to him and we parted amicably.

Alas, next morning I was met by one of my partners who had been on call the previous night and who had twice been asked to visit because the pain had recurred.

'Do you think', he asked, 'that he might be cooking up an appendix?' With some dread I retraced my steps later that morning and saw husband (and wife) again. I tried to convince myself that everything was well but there was minimal tenderness in the right iliac fossa. I swallowed hard and told them that I would have to send him to a surgical ward as I could not now exclude appendicitis. There was a brief silence before his wife poured forth a stream of invective about my previous reassurance and cast some doubts on my ability as diagnostician. I tried to point out, unfortunately in vain, that if her husband was suffering from appendicitis it was still in its very early stages and thus diagnosis was difficult.

I telephoned the duty house surgeon, who had been qualified for as long as six weeks, and his attitude was disdainful. 'I thought you GPs would know all about appendicitis,' he exclaimed, 'as it is the most common surgical emergency. Still, I suppose you'd better send him in and I'll try and sort it out for you.'

Two days later he was discharged symptom- and operation-free. His pain had settled on admission and the consultant surgeon had decided nothing needed to be done. This was in itself remarkable as he was a surgeon of the old style, always immaculately dressed in striped trousers. He was about six feet tall and had a balding ovoid head; courteous and competent, he would operate on anybody for anything, and usually did. When his discharge letter arrived it contained the memorable sentence 'He may have had a bowel inflammation or some other intra-abdominal glandular complaint.'

When I received the letter I called again on the family. The hostility that had marked my last visit was gone and the wife was smiling and happy.

'I never doubted your original diagnosis,' she lied, 'after all it was your partner who suggested that my husband's appendix was involved.'

Again I tried to explain the problems of diagnosing non-specific abdominal pain and this time I felt that my words fell on less stony ground. We parted the best of friends despite the fact that I stood on one of their cats in the rather dark hallway. (At least cats run away. I once stood on a black and tan Dachshund on a black and tan carpet and received a multitude of black and tan bruises after the dog savaged my ankle.)

As the days of that warm summer lengthened into an only slightly less warm autumn (remember this was some years ago) I forgot this couple as other, more urgent, medical and social problems occupied my waking and, sometimes sleeping, hours. In short, life appeared to be drifting along uneventfully. How wrong I was. One evening after a fairly heavy day on call a familiar commanding voice on the 'phone required my presence as the Headmaster was 'in agony' with his usual abdominal complaint.

My dictionary defines 'agony' as 'intense bodily or mental

suffering: pangs of death' and I suspect that this word is the one that is the most inappropriately over-used in the whole of the English language. Most of those unfortunates described to me as being 'in agony' are usually in any state from having a splinter in the finger to diarrhoea, but they are very seldom suffering and never anywhere remotely near the pangs of death. Because of this I did not rush to the house but instead finished my cup of tea.

I arrived at the house to find a grim-faced wife, arms folded purposefully, waiting for me at the front door. That I had taken about fifteen minutes less on this occasion than the time that I had abandoned my meal was of no relevance to her. She pointed wordlessly up the stairs to the familiar bedroom and followed me up, equally mute.

The Headmaster did not look as well as he usually did. He was lying with a slight layer of sweat on his upper lip and looked even more meek and inoffensive than usual. The pain was more severe on this occasion, according to his spokeswoman, and he had been in terrible suffering – and she had had two children and knew all about suffering. His temperature was slightly raised at 99° (sorry I mean 37.2°) but again there were no outstanding physical signs. I came face to face with cowardice – and lost. I sent him back to into hospital where he remained for forty-eight hours during which time nothing was done to him (I believe this is called 'observation') and he was returned to the bosom of his family.

On this occasion, however, he remained vaguely unwell with bouts of intermittent pain. I visited regularly but no clinical, biochemical or radiological abnormalities were discovered. I suffered the growing criticisms of his wife as stoically as those from her husband. One evening I was again summoned urgently during my evening meal (why do emergencies, i.e., 'come straight away' calls inevitably interrupt essential physiological functions?) but on this occasion I was bidden to attend by a male voice which was not wholly familiar but which, I was certain, I had heard before. I arrived at the house where the full might of the family were assembled, and waiting for me in the hall were wife, son, daughter and daughter's tiro journalist paramour.

'It's bloody disgraceful' said the son, 'that my father should have had so much suffering. You doctors aren't accountable enough, that's the trouble. Something will have to change. Now get your bloody finger out and cure him, or else I'll report you to a higher authority.'

The daughter joined in the onslaught. 'This is typical of your collusion of anonymity' she said (she, too, had obviously read Balint). 'I shall get Rudi' pointing to her boyfriend 'to expose you in his paper.'

I resisted, admittedly with great personal sacrifice, the temptation to respond in kind and murmured, 'Perhaps I had better see the patient.' He was lying, as inoffensively as ever, in bed and was very apologetic about my reception committee. Again he described the pain but, as before, there was nothing to find on examination. I went downstairs to face my inquisitors who were scathing about the abilities of my colleagues and myself to cure their father who was 'obviously seriously ill – and you don't care about it!'

I suspect that most family doctors have faced such situations at some stage in their careers. Patients, and more particularly their relatives, are frightened by illness and behave in an aggressive manner. Nevertheless, I was disconcerted by the accusation about lack of care as I had seen the patient frequently over the previous weeks. However, I said that I would arrange a visit the following day with a surgical specialist from the local hospital, assuring them, after a heated and offensive interjection from the son, that this would *not* be a private consultation but would be carried out under the NHS.

I thought of asking our most recently appointed surgeon to call. After all, he wore sports jackets and flannel trousers instead of the more formal garb of the senior surgeon and this might have appeased the son's radical social thoughts. However, I felt that clinical continuity was more important and arranged to meet with the surgeon under whom the Headmaster had been admitted some weeks before.

We met at the house: I arrived in my elderly Fiat and he in his new Jaguar. The son was in fine voice.

'I hope' he said to the surgeon, 'that you can sort my father out as this fellow here' pointing at me, 'obviously doesn't have a clue.'

We proceeded to the bedroom and the consultation was as uneventful as it was unproductive. The surgeon said he could find nothing seriously amiss, reassured the Headmaster that he did not have appendicitis and suggested that I tried an intestinal antispasmodic (I'd already used nearly every one listed in *MIMS*.) At his car, he turned to me and said 'What a charming man. Pity about his family though. I suppose they didn't have the right sort of nanny when they were younger'. And he was serious!

The second opinion appeared to allay the family's anxieties and they actually allowed the patient to visit me during the next few weeks in order to collect another prescription for his antispasmodic.

A month or so later I went on holiday for a few days, preferring the company of my wife and teenage daughter to the imprecations of the Headmaster's wife. The rest of his family had by then returned to their homes in the Deep South.

On my return to work I was greeted by my senior partner who told me that he had, one Saturday afternoon, been called to see the Headmaster and had arranged an emergency admission to the Surgical Unit where his acutely inflamed, about to perforate, appendix was removed. There was no other pathology discovered. He had a stormy convalescence, complicated by a deep vein thrombosis and his family had stormed the surgery in my absence threatening to sue me and report me to 'the BMA!'

My relationship with the family was never the same afterwards and eventually they left the practice to join a rival partnership just down the road from our surgery.

However, just before they left the list that Christmas the Headmaster had an appointment with me – he needed a repeat prescription of his warfarin – and diffidently produced a parcel wrapped in Christmas paper.

'You worked so hard to help me' he said quietly, 'and I would like you to have this. Remember that it was Aristotle who said that 'a plausible impossibility is always preferable to an unconvincing possibility!'

As I took the parcel from him, thanking him effusively for his kindness, I heard the sound of liquid in a bottle and knew that he had given me one of the bottles of his Highland Single Malt whisky. Joyfully, I took it home that evening and placed it with our other presents under the Christmas tree.

On Christmas morning we opened our presents as usual and I seized the Headmaster's gift eagerly, wondering whether the bottle would be from Speyside or Islay. I tore off the wrapping paper and stared at the bottle in my hand.

It contained his appendix, preserved in formalin.

JOHN HAWORTH
Carlisle

Some of my friends seem to think that low I-Q patients must be one of the hardships of general practice. But for me, the slower-witted ones come as balm to the tired mind, a lull in the remorseless doctor-patient strife. There is never that uneasy feeling that as you try to sum up the patient the converse is also going on. How much hearing time will satisfy them? How much of a 'thorough examination' are they determined to have? These questions do not arise. If they do happen to ask 'Why is it?' or 'Where could such a thing have come from?' any explanation will be accepted with respect and thanks.[14]

Just One Extra

Dr Boris Charles looked anxiously at his Vermox digital watch. Hmmm, seven fifteen. His friends would already be congregating in the Strathallan Hotel, limbering up with the first pints of the evening, back-slapping and laughing raucously. It was the Isle of Scrot Rugby Club's annual dinner.

'Just one extra, if you don't mind?' Jessie the receptionist smiled apologetically. Dr Charles grunted. What difference would another five minutes make? A folder of notes the size of a half brick thudded onto his desk. Before he could utter a worthwhile blasphemy, Mrs Mary MacNeep (an unlikely looking woman to have engendered so much verbiage) blustered in.

'I can't go on with this any longer.' 'Something's got to be done,' anticipated Dr Charles, semi-audibly. 'What?' 'I said it can't be much fun.' 'Huh. Is there any news from that specialist yet?'

He located the latest bulletin with some difficulty and scanned through the expected verdict, '. . . will not bore you by repeating details . . . lengthy history . . . hysterectomy . . . low back pain . . . cholecystectomy . . . more than fully investigated . . . could reveal nothing abnormal . . . rather intense nature . . . strong functional element . . .'. 'What's he say?' 'Well, he's sure that there's nothing seriously . . .' 'You mean I'm being neurotic?' 'Yes,' thought Dr Charles. 'No,' said Dr Charles, glancing surreptitiously at the time. 'Anyway,' she went on, 'why doesn't anybody know what causes it, this Irritable Colon, or Spastic Spleen, or whatever it's called? What am I supposed to do about it? What about a special diet? Isn't it something to do with food allergy, then?' 'No, it's nothing at all to do with your diet.' 'Well, the specialist said it is,' she interrupted, with undisguised satisfaction. 'He said it could be an allergy to milk or wheat or anything.'

At that moment Dr Charles hated her very deeply, with the sort of conviction he usually reserved for the person just ahead of him in every bank queue, with two large muslin bags of loose change and four paying-in books. He took a deep breath. 'Look, Mrs MacNeep,' he began slowly, 'pain can be triggered on any number of levels. Certainly, there might be something in your diet which makes things worse. But physical pain can also be an expression of inner tension, or dissatisfaction, or depression . . .'

One hour and ten minutes later, Mrs MacNeep was leaving the surgery. 'Well, I can't thank you enough, doctor, and nobody has ever taken the time to explain things before. I feel much happier about it all now. Good-night.' 'Good-night,' he replied weakly. He suddenly felt exhausted. The dinner would be well under way, the beer and the jokes in full flow. By the time he had been home to wash and change, it would hardly be worth the effort . . .

His thoughts were displaced by a familiar gnawing pain, deep under his breastbone. He instinctively felt in his pocket for the Milk of Magnesia tablets, and wondered again whether he should have a barium meal.

ALAN DAVIS
St Austell

The last patient is often a problem, the reason for being last may be some communication defect such as deafness or inability to speak the language, so that priority may have been given to other patients. Two studies of the strains that doctors feel when dealing with difficult patients were made by three general practitioners. One called these patients 'heartsink patients' because they evoke an overwhelming mixture of exasperation, defeat and sense of frustration which causes the heart to sink when they consult.[15] In the other study,[16] problem patients were classified as dependent clingers, entitled demanders, self-destructive deniers, manipulative help rejectors and those who had no shared language with the doctor. Little research has been carried out on the matter of difficult doctors; one type is shown on page 115.

I never knu a man yet who was allwuss watching his helth, to die enny whare near az soon as he expected to.

HENRY WHEELER SHAW/
'JOSH BILLINGS'
1818–1885.[17]

Contemplation: a memo to the Family Practitioner Committee administrator (after W.S. Gilbert)

As one day it may happen that our work needs sorting out,
   We've got our practice list – we're looking through the list
At some surgery attenders whom we well could do without,
   And who never would be missed – who never would be missed!
There's the seventeen-stone girl who swears she eats 'just like
   a bird'
The aerophagic dowager whose plaint is loudly heard,
All anorexic virgins with their dietary quirks,
And all the costive matrons whose digestion never works,
   And the hooligans who burst into your office when they're
   p****d
They'd none of them be missed – they'd none of them be
   missed.

There's the hobnail-livered veteran who 'hardly takes a drop' –
   And the whole-food herbalist – I'll take him off my list –
The neurotics whose recitals, like their bowels, never stop –
   They never would be missed – they never would be missed!
Then the corpulent executive with the apoplectic face
Whose ulcers, gout and gallstones all compete for pride of
   place,
And the child who 'never eats' but still has strength to wreck
   your room
Whose mother's haggard face portrays anxiety and gloom,
   While his father keeps demanding he should see a specialist
   –
I don't think he'd be missed – I'm sure he'd not be missed.

Chorus

And it really doesn't matter who gets taken off the list
For they'll none of them be missed – they'll none of them be
   missed!

MARIE CAMPKIN
London

9
Feedback From Patients

'Gentlemen — It may not have escaped your professional observation that there are only two classes of mankind — doctors and patients. I have had a delicacy in confessing that I belong to the patient class ever since a doctor told me that all patients were phenomenal liars, where their own symptoms were concerned'. Rudyard Kipling when he addressed medical students at the Middlesex Hospital in 1908.[18]

Medical students and doctors make better doctors if they have been ill as they see the other side. Doctors often write usefully about their experiences as patients as shown on the Personal View page of the British Medical Journal. 'Doctors as Patients — Roles Reversed' was the title of an address given by the founder father and former President of the Royal College of General Practitioners, Lord Hunt of Fawley.[19]

Fundamental Concerns

It was always known as 'Dad's Problem' and had caused me much tribulation over the years. It had been a continual distraction from matters intellectual and had frustrated a promising sporting career. It had wreaked havoc with my singing, for my upper register had been severely curtailed by the uncertainty of my base parts. Moreover, I had developed an air of concern earlier than I could have anticipated.

It still puzzles me why, after so many years, I should have decided to have something done. But decide I did, anticipating a quick, clean, painless job with minimal inconvenience. Alas, it was not to be. Somehow, the matter escalated to a formal, planned admission for the ultimate in cold surgery.

So long as the decision remained an intellectual one, the prospect caused me little worry. As a matter of fact, the whole business generated many a merry quip and much witty conversation. Friends and acquaintances who were aware of my impending appointment with fate dipped eagerly into that

vast genre of humour that is poignantly familiar to anyone
with my problem. There was rarely anything original in their
jocular conversation. Everything to be said on this subject has
been said. Many times.

As the time approached, though, I grew uneasy and felt that
people were talking about me. I began to dread, not just the
admission and operation, but hospital visitors. After all, my
complaint was hardly the stuff of which tea-time chats are
made. My son, a personnel manager in the making, counselled
me frequently. 'But think of the chocolate and grapes, dad . . .'
(can I think of anything else); 'There'll be piles of things to talk
about . . . home and that,' he finished lamely.

For days I considered which book to take in with me. A
friend of mine, a Trappist monk, fell heavily while cleaning
windows at the monastery. As he was transferred to hospital
for repair of his extensive lacerations, the Abbot slipped a book
under his blanket. It was entitled *To Heaven Through a Window*
by St Gerard Majella. I suppose my obvious choice would be
The Grapes of Wrath by Steinbeck, but I had read it. In view of
the expected treatment, perhaps a treatise on Arctic exploration may have been appropriate, but my outlook seemed bleak
enough without that. I eventually chose, in hope, *I Can't Stay
Long*, by Laurie Lee.

My wife, being somewhat devout, suggested that I should
be included that week in the Parish Sick List which was published every Sunday. I demurred. It's not that I lack faith in the
prayers of my fellow Christians. Oh no. But it is difficult to
imagine just what prayers they might say. So far as I know the
Saints and Doctors of the Church have not concerned themselves unduly with my particular problem. Holy Writ has little
to say on the subject. There were other worries too, about the
Sick List. Every Sunday, it reminds me of my failures. I do not
recall offhand anyone who, once included, ever left it, except
by one rather final route. Moreover, the curate who usually
types out the Parish Bulletin has many gifts but included in
those gifts are not spelling and typing. Misprints abound. One
poor soul had Mass said for her mother's 'Recovery from silli-
ness'. Got talked about for ages, she did. I did not dare imagine
what they might make of my infirmity.

On that fateful morning I was brightly unconcerned. I rejected my wife's offer of help with the packing. I was quite capable of doing it myself. As soon as she had left for work, I sought out all that was necessary. The pyjamas and toothbrush were easy. My dressing gown, so rarely used, had lost its cord in some long forgotten game of Cowboys and Indians. It gaped alarmingly and revealingly at the slightest movement. It was difficult to know what to put soap and things into. The only available toilet bag I could find belonged to my daughter. It was pink and fluffy and had lace trimmings. It did not seem to me to adequately represent the macho image I had of myself, but there was nothing else. I stuffed it to the bottom of the bag, out of sight.

On my way out, I looked in on my greenhouse. I looked upon the trusses of swollen red tomatoes and wondered. I snipped off the ripest and tears came into my eyes.

The grey wetness of the morning complemented my inner mood. Unconsciously, I over-asserted my own identity. With my college tie in place, wearing a tastefully monogrammed sweater and carrying a carelessly chosen light, overtly medical textbook, I walked jauntily to my fate. As I entered the ward, I became, immediately, that five-year-old boy on his first day at school so many years ago.

I tried so very hard to be the perfect, all-accepting patient, but my underlying anxiety continually revealed itself in slightly hysterical humour. Being 'clerked in' was a tense procedure. I found myself assessing the significance of every 'Mm' and 'Good' that the nurse muttered. Some questions obviously embarrassed her and I became tongue tied. Other questions I could relax with. 'Nothing to worry about on that score,' I would announce confidently. When she had finished, she fastened a small plastic bracelet to my wrist. It had my name on it.

My next visitor was the girl from the laboratory, come to take the inevitable blood test. I felt a rising panic. In my mind, I totted up quickly the number of glasses of wine I had consumed in the last few weeks and prayed that it would not show in the laboratory. I could almost hear the conversation. 'Have you seen this?' 'Oh, him. I'm not surprised.' The technician and I chatted as she drew the blood. Our talk was, at best, desultory and I tried to enliven it. My voice was curiously high-pitched and my humour flat and unoriginal. She smiled, thinly I thought, and left.

And then the long wait. It had been a long time since I had sat quietly alone for hours, with all responsibility gone. I read, then I read some more. I drank a lot of water and then went to the toilet. I combed my hair. Then I had another drink of water and went to the toilet again. I looked out of the window to a now sun-bright day. It was no distraction and, in fact, served only to exaggerate my imprisonment. Out there were people who were not in here. Some seemed to have a purpose in their lives, others were just walking about. I saw colleagues coming and going to and from the staff car park. They were talking to each other, telling funny stories and swapping anecdotes about patients. Of whom I was one.

By 7 o'clock, a long evening still lay ahead. I had not yet changed into my pyjamas, lest I lost the last vestige of my identity. Even so, my eyes still strayed frequently to the band around my wrist that told me who I was. Despite the fact that it was still only autumn, the bellringers at the nearby church were practicing 'O Come, O Come Emmanuel' – and getting the last note wrong every time. I meditated on the problems of being a new bellringer and wondered how one made a start. It seemed to me that however one started, that first bum note would resound throughout the city. I must have been emotionally fragile, for, before I knew what I was doing, I was silently weeping for apprentice bellringers. But the wrong note was repeated so often that my mood gradually changed from empathetic sadness to a great anger and, by 8.30 p.m., I was ready to form a society for the abolition of bellringers. Especially apprentices.

I was aware that some medical activity that night was inevitable. I could not bear to define it in my own mind, but I knew it would be pretty basic. All the old jokes surfaced from my memory and failed to amuse me. I debated within myself how best to greet the nurse and her stainless steel trolley. 'Hello. Are you a friend or an enema?' No. My hysterical laughter would betray me. Besides, she's probably heard it before. Best be formal. 'Good evening, nurse, I await your pleasure.' P'raps I'll forego the last bit. And any comment on the weather would be bound to be misconstrued. I was, in the event, as formal as can be expected under the circumstances and took the administration almost without qualm. Alas, I found that it was not only my memory that failed to retain. My feeling of inadequacy deepened.

By now I was totally unsure and indecisive. Switching on the television took a great effort of will and much looking over my shoulder. It was not worth it for all that appeared was an electronic snowstorm. The sound was clear enough though. While fiddling with the controls, a benign and reassuring anaesthetist visited me and gave me 4 mg of lorazepam. Full of trepidation at their likely effect, I took them, rushed to clean my teeth, changed and leapt into bed, expecting to be poleaxed any minute. Nothing happened. Or perhaps something did, for when the night nurse came in, I asked about the television and explained the problem. I would not have dared to do so before the lorazepam. He brought me another set. The picture was fine, but the sound was distorted, no matter what we did. I settled for both on at the same time, though changing channels was a complex procedure and the two sets were not always compatible. This confusion, combined with the increasing effects of the drug, produced some curious and bizzare effects.

So far, I have not mentioned my multifocals. Very few people do, I find. There are times when the claims for their excellence and convenience seem to me to be overstated. I admit that they are fine for watching television while sitting square on, in a chair. But lying down, with one eye necessarily above the other, eliminates clear vision in all parts of the picture apart from the central one square centimetre. And anyway they pressed painfully into my head.

Gradually, I became calmer and more relaxed. I began to prepare myself mentally for the morrow, for I would be going over the top. In a manner of speaking.

I remember little of THE DAY other than smiling faces, jocular rejoinders and no pain. My son tells me that I had all the advantages of being drunk but none of the disadvantages. I am assured I was convivial, though a trifle uninhibited. Those operating gowns do little to restrain one's inhibitions – or anything else, for that matter.

I think one of my trainees visited me. I can vaguely recall a stubbled, tieless man with intense eyes expounding on the novel he had left me. It was all about the Devil visiting Moscow once. I believed him and took it as read. It was the next day when, with a nearly normal mind, my fundamental concern became apparent. Gradually that concern grew to a painful obsession. There was no avoiding the dénouement. I strode manfully to that small room for my moment of truth. Ten painful minutes later, I returned, aware that another milestone had been passed.

The headline in the sunday paper announced that another union had suffered sequestration of their assets. I knew how they felt.

Overall, I think that my visitors had a pretty raw deal. My room was not the place to be if you wanted stimulating conversation, spiced with heart-rending, blood-curdling tales of the sharp end of the National Health Service. In fact, my news had about it a repetitive inconsequence that bored even me. Nor could I evince anything other than disinterest in the news from home. I had hoped that the natural euphoria that follows the completion of a trial would be sufficient to carry my visitors along, but it wasn't. I was aware of a feeling of disappointment in the air. Several remarked, somewhat sharply I thought, on how well I looked. There were one or two who had, I am certain, a similar problem to my own. I could tell by their sheepish entrance, the obvious discomfort of their posture and, most of all by the yellow pallor of their faces as I described again the technical details of the operation.

There was no doubt that the turning point in my hospital stay was the coming of the lucozade. You can't argue with lucozade. It gives a chap status and I was, at last, a proper patient. People began to pay me proper respect and asked me how I was feeling. Chocolate and magazines were not long in their coming and a rather fine beaujolais enlivened the menu no end. I became relaxed with the staff and joked and grumbled as the season declared. The routine of the hospital day dominated my every thought and action. Each event was keenly anticipated and timed. There was a major crisis on the fourth day. For reasons I could not understand, the spirit did not move me as easily as it might have done and the subsequent delay resulted in my missing the morning paper round. I panicked. What could I do between coffee and lunch? The day crumbled about me. I sank into a profound depression. So deep was my despair that I read the Sunday papers again.

Later that day, the surgeon came to see me to ask how I was. Suddenly and miraculously all my symptoms disappeared. No longer did I suffer from all those terrible afflictions I had endured through my slough of despond. 'Absolutely splendid' was I in answer to his every query. I was terrified in case he kept me in any longer or, heaven forbid, did the job again.

The great return home was a little disappointing. An important badge of illness in our house has always been the inalienable right to lie on the settee if you are feeling in any way poorly. This right takes precedence over all others, including the strength of emotion generated by mother's varicose veins. But I could not get comfortable and those damned multifocals didn't focus properly. I resigned my rights and sat on a chair, losing all presence in so doing. The other major problem was more subtle. Illness needs to exist in its own right to be properly enjoyed. There is not room in any family for more than one illness at a time. Certainly this is the case in our house. Imagine my chagrin, therefore, when Grandma went off it as soon as I got home. She even had the doctor calling to see her. Never noticed me he didn't, even though I'd got a special short dressing gown for my convalescence. I went back to work early.

Formerly the successful doctor was said to need three things: a top hat to give him authority, a paunch to give him dignity, and piles to give him an anxious expression.

I have often wondered since then why I had it done at that particular time. I suspect I needed to try myself out, to see how I could cope with the gentle ripple of symptoms that heralds the onset of middle age. Well, I did survive and I am reassured. Actually, it wasn't that bad.

I think I'll have that hernia done next year.

RONALD MULROY
Wakefield

And patient feedback is interesting and helpful, as from this rather neurotic patient:

Dynamite Ivy

So, you want to hear about my 'tummy troubles'? If yes, then listen carefully but don't sit gormless on your bum – just put your feet up and relax – blast your gases away – keep up the 'bowel club' tradition. My mother always quotes an engraving on an old friend's grave: 'Wherever you may be, let your wind go free, for holding it was the death of me'.

Let me give you a short family 'istry – at least that is what all doctors ask. Poor souls! I feel sorry for them. I would not like to have their job even as a pensioner.

I will start with a clean plate — no garlic, no senokot. Let me look up my note-book. Don't get excited – it is not a porn story! Nor is it a video nasty!

Call me Ivy, although my name by natural birth is Topsy Shufflebottom. My mother gave me that name because she said I was born with 'bottoms up'. My originals were Vikings. My family is nicknamed 'bowel family' – perhaps because they were always obscened with their bowels. My mother taught me to keep my 'tickles' clean – always. I am slightly erotic [neurotic]! That is why they have put my picture and account of my bowels in so many medical papers. You must read them up for your examinations. You cannot mistake it – even if your antique memory fails you.

I am middle-aged and happily married three times. My present husband is a gentleman, he never touches me. We go our own way because we always crash. That is why we go on separate holidays. My husband is on the social club because he can't stand on both his legs, but he enjoys a tot and a flutter on the horses. Unfortunately, the horses don't like him – he always loses! Mind you, he tries hard but then has the 'runs'. He is a very caring man. Every morning he pokes tablets in my mouth before he goes out for a walk with the dog.

My mother is a God-frightened soul. She goes to church regularly but cannot stay there long – has to go to the loo – she cannot keep her 'secrets' long. My grandmother's bowels are still in the medical college museum. I have seen them in a glass jar, I wonder why they look black. Could she have had coloured or gipsy blood in her?

My father is dead. Oh, he was a strapping lad – went to the Windmill Theatre and local regularly, drank like a rhino! He didn't like to have any worries, he borrowed money from my mother, but treated the boys with free drinks regularly at the local. Mind you, in his latter days be became a Scrooge and stopped spending a penny for anybody. My mother says that this was because his lines got blocked with cauliflower like growths. He was found dead in bed. Fowl play was suspected as he did not leave a note about the cause of his death.

Where was I? Sorry for wandering away! You see I told you I was erotic! I got carried away with my family tree. Yes, I was going to tell you about my personal body bowels.

I got my bowel trouble about a year ago – I can tell you the exact date – it was the day when a bearded man exposed himself to me. I felt sick – actually vomited and then got the 'runs'. Since then I get loud rumblings and thunders in my tummy from time to time. My tummy blows up like a balloon and then 'gushings' come out. My grandson of six thinks I have a baby inside me. He pats my tummy and asks 'Granny, when is the baby coming out? He is groaning. He doesn't like it in there, he wants to come out'. I feel so bashful!

One day I said enough is enough. I decided to see my GP. It

is so difficult to get appointment with him. It is easier to see the Queen than my doctor. It is the dragon – his receptionist one has to climb over. She gave me an appointment for the following week. I could not wait that long so I contacted the 'Help Line'. They advised me either to call my GP for a visit or go to accident and emergency department of my local hospital. I didn't want to call my GP because he thinks I am 'nuts' and waste his time. Casualty hospital advised me to see a specialist through my GP. Thank heavens, I could see my GP the next day as another patient cancelled her appointment with him.

My GP is a tall handsome man. I would not change him for anything. When I went to see him first time for my bowels, I dressed up like a doll with my best clothes and perfume. Of course I had got my hair permed that very day with highlights. I also took my brolly, jug of coffee and toilet roll – in case...

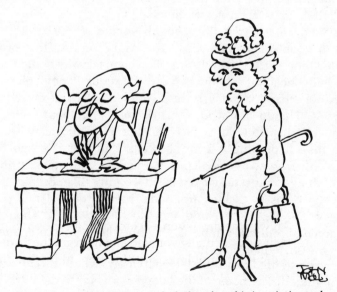

The doctor said hallo but never looked up from his inscription pad

The receptionist gave me a dirty look when I walked in but I didn't care. Very soon the light outside my doctor's room flashed. I thought the doctor was in distress (and I will not blame him for that). So I ran to the receptionist and pointed out the flashing light. She gave me a cold look just as you do to a dog and asked me to go in. The doctor said hallo but never looked up from his inscription pad. I felt terribly disappointed. I started to tell him about my bowels when I was suddenly seized with gripping pain and wind in my stomach – then a huge blast of wind thundered out from my lower end – I felt so ashamed but I couldn't help it. It was so sudden and loud! He looked shocked and went deathly pale and stopped making notes. He thought it was a bomb! Then suddenly he sprang to life and scrambled to the door to open it. He gave me a quick piscission and I cashed it from a confounded chemist who gave me funny looks.

When I visited my GP second time, I saw him red in the face, agitated and pacing about in his consulting room while talking to me. Immediately he arranged an appointment on the telephone for me to see the specialist told me that I might have to go into hospital for investigations.

I did not like to go to the hospital. Nor did my husband want me to. I don't blame him. He has been no good since they prostrated him. Besides, would I be allowed to take my budgie and cat to the hospital? My husband would certainly not look after them. Perhaps social services would do it I murmured to myself. Then a bright idea struck me! How about seeing a homeopath who would give me 'natural' medicines without the fuss of probing into my bowels. Naturally, I asked the homeopath how his medicines worked and how these primitive things crept into a civilised country like Britain. He explained his medicines are made from nature, plants, soil, sea-weeds etc. How could you do that I asked? Then he chanted his mumbo jumbo of 'Like cures like'. That completely put me off. What rubbish!

I was admitted to hospital. I felt trembly like a pig ready to be slaughtered. The name of the hospital is a blur to me – I think it was called 'Cheery or Cherry something'; it was far from it. As I entered the gate of the hospital, I saw a sign board saying – danger, don't go round the bend.

I passed the wards named 'Faith', 'Hope' and 'Victory'. I lingered with a fond hope for being admitted into one of them but they decided to put me in 'Patience' – 'trying to shut me up' I said to myself with paranoid feelings. My gloomy forebodings began to evaporate when I saw the bright and clean atmosphere of the ward but I developed a 'relapse' when I saw the sister. She growled and walked like a sergeant-major. When she sat in a chair, she looked ferocious like a dinosaur with a big frame and large eyes darting to and fro – marking every event occurring in the ward. The patients had a frozen resigned look.

The routine was to wake us up every morning at about 5 a.m. (not that I slept much mind you, what with all the ramblings and moanings going on all night). Nurses would go round taking temperatures, giving medicines except bedpans which I needed the most. They are sadists!

When the morning came, medical students and junior doctors came to us all – one by one in turn. They asked such intimate questions – including our past and family! Other silly questions were 'How many times do you go to the toilet?' I replied, that is my private affair. Besides, I don't keep a diary of my visits to the loo.

A coloured student asked me whether I had blood in my stools and if yes whether the blood was bright red or dark? I laughed and replied 'To the best of my knowledge, all bloods have the same colour. Besides, I do not stick my nose into the toilet seat to see if there is any blood'. What a silly bloke.

Then these students prodded and poked and interfered with me all over. 'Have you finished' I screamed? 'I am bursting to go to the loo.' They are such a rough lot! They think they have a license to play with your body once they have worn a white coat. Then the cheeky devils discussed my case near my bed. One of them said I had irritating bowel – no wonder – with all my gas and electricity bills. A Chinese bloke said that I had some sort of infection – possibly giada or 'see-look'. I did not know what 'see' or 'look' were doing. Then a coloured student blurted out Crow's disease. I have never eaten a crow in my life. A white bloke said it could be a neopatism, another bloke thought my tyroid gland was running too fast and had to be halted. A silly looking lady student suggested I had dysititis with divers, what a bloody cheek. Then another mumbled 'culitis' whatever that means. They could not agree on anything. They left me terrified and palpitating.

Later in the day the specialist came. Everything went deathly silent but he was very nice and gentle. He gave me a thorough check-up from top to bottom. Why aren't all doctors Specialists? At least they will then know what they are doing. Then he arranged for my blood tests and stool tests. Collecting stools was nauseating – to say the least. Then the specialist passed a long telescope through my lower guts – it was so embarrassing! He said he could see everything clearly and there was nothing of note – I don't know what he meant! He told me he took a bite from my bowels. I am sure it must be awful! The worst was still to come – it was what they call Barium Enema. I don't know who invented it. They tossed me and mucked me about so much that I felt like bashing the X-ray specialists' head. I collapsed while they were taking my pictures.

During this collapse my soul flew out of my body. You don't believe me when I say this. You think I am crazy. No, it is true! I could see them thumping my chest and blowing into my mouth. One of them shouted 'she's gone'. I smiled and travelled fast through a dark tunnel. And there at the end of it was light and my grandmother. She murmured 'You will be alright. It is not time yet for you to come here. Don't allow these fools to muck you about. Stop taking too many tablets. It is not necessary to have your bowels open daily. Stop worrying about things. Take All Bran.' And then suddenly I was woken up by a smiling face asking me. 'How are you feeling Mrs Robinson?'

I have come back to the ward lying prostate and praying to God which I have never done before. Nothing has changed. I am still blown out with wind, have rumblings up and down my tummy and occasional runs. However, for the first time in my life I have felt the presence of angels around me and love of merciful God. I feel I am in a space-shuttle propelled by gas bobbing me up and down!

I bet you do not understand what I am talking about! Perhaps because you cannot understand humans or even animals! Maybe you are a sexist! Did you say you are a GP?

Maybe, you call yourself a doctor – but you are not as good as some doctors who can see patients' problems through their bosoms or under their feet. My priest had already warned me to be wary of bloody caretakers or undertakers – whatever you're called – like you!

Listen carefully – if you want to be a 'proper' doctor. I wanted kids, I could not have them. They told me I had blocked tubes because of some infection. I tried to purge my germs away with vodka and whisky. These stayed in my body and soul – I grew rotten. Then I tried my friend's tablets given to her by her doctor. They nearly killed me!

I bet you still haven't a clue about my illness! My grandmother knew it. Her words keep on ringing in my ears, 'stop worrying, stop taking too many tablets. You will be alright.'

A.A. SHAIKH
London

10
Tales of the Unexpected

It is an old maxim of mine that when you
have excluded the impossible, whatever
remains, however improbable, must be the
truth

SIR ARTHUR CONAN DOYLE
In *The Adventures of Sherlock Holmes*[20]

A Breath of Air

Dr Waterfall entered his surgery with unusual briskness for
a Monday morning. He looked forward to the comfortable
routines of his own consulting room after the exotic atmosphere of the weekend course that he had just attended.

He was still not sure what had attracted him to that particular course. 'Intra-Familial Psychodynamics and the Art of
Manipulating the Environment' was not a subject close to his
heart; perhaps the very obscurity of the title had in some per-
verse way aroused his interest.

Against his expectations, he had quite enjoyed the
weekend. He had met some strange people and been introduced to some amusing but entirely abstract ideas that could
not possibly be applied to the stolid patients of his own practice.

He looked around his room and was reassured to find that it
was just as he had left it on the Friday night. He glanced at the
list of patients due to see him that morning, and recognised
every name. He was long reconciled to the fact that for many
of them there would be no cure; he had accepted the role of
guide to these unfortunates, pointing them along their roads
in something like the right direction. He was quite content
with this function, quite happy to leave the more dramatic
episodes of the practice, whenever possible, to his young
partners.

He settled down into his chair, leant across the desk, and pressed the button that summoned his first patient. A few seconds later there was a hesitant knock on the door and a small thin-faced man carrying a plastic carrier-bag slid sideways into the room. Dr Waterfall turned towards him. 'Good morning Mr Perkins. Do sit down.' He waved towards the empty chair. 'How are you getting on? Are the pains any better?'

Mr Perkins stood holding the carrier-bag awkwardly in front of him, unsure what to do with it. The doctor, who had seen the bag a hundred times before, now suddenly recognised it for the first time as a blatant emblem of his patient's widower status. Mr Perkins then leant the bag carefully against the wall and sat down on the front edge of the proffered seat. He looked up at the doctor with a face that wore an expression of deep suffering bravely endured.

'It's no better at all,' he said, shaking his head slowly. 'It's just like a knife. Here.' He placed the flat of his right hand on his abdomen and rotated it slowly in a clockwise direction.

Dr Waterfall looked at the moving hand with an expression of concern which deepened as he turned to the bulging folder of notes that his patient had accumulated. 'Let's see, now,' he said. 'We were doing some more investigations, were'nt we.' He rifled through the mass of papers. 'That's right,' Mr Perkins said. 'I had to swallow that tube again. Have you got the results yet?' 'Yes, here we are,' the doctor said, glancing briefly at a report, then handing it across to Mr Perkins. 'As you can see, everything is absolutely normal. No ulcers or cancers or anything else to worry about.' Mr Perkins displayed less than total joy at this news. 'So why am I still having the pain?' he asked. The doctor sighed. 'Have you really no idea at all what brings it on? Are you quite sure it doesn't come on after food? Or when you walk fast?' 'I'm sorry, but it doesn't, doctor. Like I said, it comes on at any time. Just like a knife.'

As Dr Waterfall sat back to search for new phrases of comfort, he was suddenly aware that alien thoughts were entering his mind, that unexpected sentences were waiting to be spoken. He sat forward again, peered at his patient, and decided to give these words their freedom.

'Tell me, Mr Perkins,' he said, listening in astonishment to his own words, 'do you ever experience bouts of almost uncontrollable rage and anger? Do you feel aggression so fierce that you wonder how you can possibly restrain yourself from acts of extreme violence?'

Mr Perkins's jaw dropped as he stared in bewilderment at these questions. 'I'm sorry but I don't,' he managed to whisper. 'No, nothing like that at all.' 'Then we have discovered your trouble,' the doctor said triumphantly. 'All that aggression is bottled up inside you, along with a whole bagful of frustrated sexual urges I've no doubt. No wonder it feels like a knife. Just there.' He pointed an accusing finger in the direction of Mr Perkins's midriff.

Mr Perkins gazed in disbelief at this latest opinion on his condition. Dr Waterfall sat back to recover from this amazing speech; he suspected that Mr Perkins had no idea what he was talking about, but he felt that he had ventured quite far enough for one day. 'Well, you just think about it,' he said. 'Keep on with the tablets and come back again in a fortnight.' Mr Perkins, relieved that the consultation was over, scuttled from the room without a backward glance. When the door was closed Dr Waterfall sat still for a while, contemplating a whole new world of medicine that was opening up before him. Then he pressed the buzzer and prepared himself to meet the next victim of inappropriate emotional adaptation.

He stood up when Mrs Robb entered. Her plump cheeks carried their usual bland smile that, as he now realised, expressed the sorrow of bereavement, but also managed to suggest that the world is not such a bad place after all. Evidence of the success of her three previous marriages was displayed on the fingers of the hand that she lifted to cover her mouth as she produced a genteel burp. 'Pardon me,' she said coyly. She sat down, arranging herself carefully on the chair.

Before Dr Waterfall could speak there was a timid knock on the door; as it opened a few inches Mr Perkins face was to be seen outside. 'I'm very sorry to trouble you, doctor,' he mumbled. 'But I left my bag behind. On the floor there.'

The doctor reached down for the bag; he was about to return it to its owner when yet again a new idea entered his consciousness. 'Mr Perkins,' he said. 'Could you take a seat in the waiting room for a minute. I'd like a word with you before you go.' He handed the bag out through the door: Mr Perkins clutched it and hurried away.

When he had gone, Dr Waterfall turned his attention back to Mrs Robb. 'And how is the hiatus hernia behaving?' 'Doctor, are you quite sure that's what the trouble is?' she asked. 'Oh, yes, of course, absolutely typical,' he answered, but his mind was elsewhere as he listened with apparent sympathy to the vivid descriptions of Mrs Robb's heartburn, and to the specimen eructations that she offered uninvited for his consideration.

As she rose to leave, the doctor asked casually, 'By the way, do you have any difficulty getting up to the surgery? It must be too far for you to walk.' 'Yes, and it can be a long wait for the bus. I get a taxi if the weather's bad.' Her smile took on a shade of sadness. 'I should have learnt to drive years ago. My last husband wanted to teach me.' 'Well, perhaps I can be of some help to you there,' he said. He called Mr Perkins back into the room. 'Do you know Mrs Robb?' he asked. Mr Perkins looked suspiciously at her and shook his head. 'You pass Mrs Robb's house on your way here,' the doctor continued, 'and she has trouble getting on to the buses. Do you think you could give her a lift home?' 'Yes, alright,' Mr Perkins said, without enthusiasm. 'And remember, I want to see you both again a fortnight today.'

After the door had closed behind them, he sat back with a pleasurable glow of satisfaction. He had just started to manipulate the environment.

Over the next few weeks, he observed a subtle change in the couple. They still complained as much as ever of their symptoms, insisting that there was no sign of any improvement; but their manner of complaining had altered. They seemed less convinced of the overwhelming importance of their symptoms, which now appeared to be moving away from the centre of their lives.

Enquiries of his staff revealed that the couple always arrived together now for their appointments, and were quite cheerful at the reception desk. They had been seen out shopping together, wheeling a shared trolley around the supermarket. Then one day Mrs Robb admitted with a flashing smile that her pains were much improved, although her flatulence was unstaunched. A few weeks later, Mr Perkins confessed that his sharp knife was now no more than an occasional dull ache in his belly. Dr Waterfall declared them cured. 'Your progress has been quite spectacular; I don't need to see you again,' he told them, separately. 'You know where I am if you want me.' They each thanked him gratefully for the cure that he wrought. He looked out of the window a few minutes later, and felt a surge of pride when he saw them driving away happily together. He began a mental search of his files for other unfortunate couples whom he might be able to help in this dramatic fashion.

About six months later he received a letter from the couple, announcing their forthcoming marriage. They were deeply thankful that he had brought them together, and hoped they would be spared to enjoy a reasonable period of happiness with each other. They would be living in Mrs Robb's house. Would the doctor look in and see them any time he was passing in the course of his rounds?

Dr Waterfall visited them several times over the next months, admiring each time the success of the marriage that he had created. The new Mrs Perkins was completely absorbed in providing the comforts of home for her husband. There was no mention of pains now, and the eructations that sometimes still occurred were ignored by all as an inevitable but trivial fact of life.

Mr Perkins said little at these visits, but he looked a different man. The shape of his face had changed; the deep furrows on his forehead had been smoothed away by the tender care of his new wife, and the hollows of his cheeks had filled out to gently convex hillocks. He sat back, enfolded by a brocaded armchair, while she attended to his needs. He looked a happy man.

It was some nine months later that Mr Perkins returned to the surgery. The vague unease the doctor had felt at the sight of his name on the list seemed quite unjustified when Mr Perkins entered his room. The man did not look ill; no doubt he had some trivial problem.

'Come in and sit down, Mr Perkins. What can I do for you?' Mr Perkins looked slightly guilty. 'It's nothing very much,' he said. 'I've just had a few of those pains come back again.' Dr Waterfall hid his disappointment. 'There's probably some good reason for it,' he said. 'A little stress perhaps. Trouble with the tax man? That sort of thing?' Mr Perkins looked thoughtfully down at the floor, then shook his head. 'No. Nothing like that at all.' 'I'd better have a look at you then. Jump up onto the couch.' Dr Waterfall examined him carefully but found nothing to account for the return of the pains. 'Perhaps you've been overeating,' he said. 'I know your wife is a wonderful cook. I'm sure it will settle down in a day or two if you take things quietly.'

But the pain did not settle down; it grew steadily worse over the following weeks. Mr Perkins described it now as a twisting griping pain that clamped down on his guts every few hours; Mrs Perkins tearfully confirmed how he lay on his bed clutching a hot water bottle, groaning in agony and praying for his Lord to take him.

Dr Waterfall was baffled; his usually effective remedies were no help at all to his patient. The urgent tests he arranged did not show the cause of the illness. Mr Perkins by now had completely lost his appetite and grew weaker every day; he took to his bed, where he lay withdrawn in between the spasms of his suffering.

Throughout all his trouble, his wife's behaviour was beyond criticism. On Dr Waterfall's visits to the house she was to be seen bustling up and down the stairs carrying a tempting dish or a hot water bottle or clean sheets and pyjamas; and always on her face was a faintest hint of the smile of a willing martyr. The doctor avoided her eyes when she showed him out of the house; he had no answer to the question that he knew they would ask him.

The consultant physician invited by Dr Waterfall to see the patient was equally baffled. Mr Perkins was now so weak that he could only raise his legs an inch or two from the sheets before they fell back, powerless.

'I'll have him in hospital for some more tests,' he told Dr Waterfall. 'He is a very sick man.' He looked significantly over his glasses. 'We must exclude – um – toxic substances, of course.'

But Mr Perkins refused to leave his home. 'I'm alright where I am,' he whispered. 'No one could look after me better than my dear wife.' 'I want him here as long as I can manage him,' his wife said bravely. 'Unless there's anything you can really do for him in the hospital.'

The physician was reluctant. 'I suppose we could do the tests from home,' he said. 'Alright. But if he gets any worse he'll have to come in at once.'

The report on the tests came through a few days later; there was no sign of any poison in the specimens that had been sent to the hospital. Dr Waterfall rang the house to say he would call on them that afternoon to discuss the next step. When he arrived he found Mrs Perkins struggling to lift her husband up from the bedroom floor; he had foolishly tried to stand up unaided, although he must have known his legs were completely unable to support even the dwindling weight of his wasting body.

The doctor lifted him easily back into his bed. 'That settles it,' he said. 'I'm going to fix a hospital bed for you. I'll ring you later with the details.'

Mr Perkins shook his head feebly, but the doctor pretended not to notice; Mrs Perkins dropped her gaze in grudging consent.

He hurried off to his evening surgery, during which he made the arrangements for the admission. He decided to call in to his patient on the way home to check that he had recovered from the effects of his fall. He let himself in through the back door of the house. The kitchen was empty. A radio was playing music loudly upstairs. He walked through the hall and, turning at the foot of the staircase, looked upwards. Mrs Perkins was standing on the landing at the top of the straight flight of stairs. He watched her profile as she manipulated the contents of a tray which lay on a small table. She did not hear or see him.

He was about to call up to her, but stifled the words as he saw a shadow moving on the landing. Then Mr Perkins was standing there, firm and upright, behind his wife's back. As the doctor watched, astounded, Mr Perkins advanced slowly towards his wife. The radio drowned any noise he made. His eyes were staring intently ahead, and his hands were held, fingers clawed, in front of him.

In the next moment Perkins sprang at his wife. The doctor let out a great roar and bounded up the stairs. Mrs Perkins screamed, there was a confused scuffle, and the tray clattered down the stairway. Mrs Perkins was left clutching the bannister rail. Perkins let go of her at the sight of the doctor, and lay cringing on the landing.

The doctor led Mrs Perkins to the sofa downstairs and left her with a glass of brandy. Upstairs again, Mr Perkins lay shivering on the landing. He looked shiftily at the doctor.

'I must have stumbled against her,' he muttered. But the truth had dawned on Dr Waterfall. 'Perkins, I can hardly believe this. All this illness is a sham, a hunger-strike. To give you an alibi when your wife was found dead at the foot of the stairs?' Mr Perkins sat up. 'You couldn't prove that,' he said sulkily. 'But why? You were so happy together.'

Mr Perkins climbed weakly to his feet and faced the doctor. 'Oh yes, we were happy enough at first,' he said. 'But then her belching got on my nerves. All day and all night – it never stopped – it drove me mad. Can you understand that? I couldn't take any more.' He paused, then gave the doctor a twisted smile. 'So I took your advice.' 'My advice?' 'Yes. You told me to be more aggressive.' 'Oh my God! So I did.' The doctor felt faint and leant against the bannister. There was a long silence before he spoke again.

'Considering all the implications, and if your wife agrees,' the doctor said eventually, 'I will take this matter no further. Provided you promise never to do anything like that again.' 'I'm sorry,' was the reply, 'but I can only promise that if you can stop her belching.' Dr Waterfall raised his eyes to the ceiling. 'You drive a hard bargain,' he said.

Mrs Perkins was still sobbing downstairs. It took all the doctor's powers of diplomacy to explain to her the reason for the assault. As he examined her under the pretext of checking for injuries, he was astonished to find extreme tenderness in the region of her gall bladder.

Months later, Mrs Perkins attended the surgery for the final check-up after her operation; Mr Perkins carried her shopping basket for her.

She beamed at the doctor across the desk. 'I feel so much better without my gall bladder,' she said. 'And I don't pass any wind at all now.'

Her husband looked down at the floor with a contented smile on his face. He took his wife's arm as they left the room. When they had gone, Dr Waterfall sat deep in thought for a few moments. Then he searched his desk and found the list of weekend courses for the coming year. 'That will do nicely,' he said out loud, putting a large tick against his chosen subject: 'Basic Symptoms and Signs in Gastroenterology'.

ERIC WILSON
Stourbridge

The Rolling Stones

It was a beautiful spring day. Daffodils, crocuses, lambs, all that stuff. The fact that it was spring is totally irrelevant to the story. Molly was home. She had had her gall-bladder removed. After years of frightful flatulence, she looked forward to wind-free days. She wouldn't miss that dreadful pain either, that terrible colic that gripped her abdomen and made her vomit. She thought wistfully that the touch of jaundice had suited her. Pity it made her eyes yellow too, but her teeth did look pearly white in contrast. She had a nice thin silvery scar. Neat and tidy, she thought, as she patted it gently with baby powder. Not like Mrs Johnson's huge wide track winding all over her fat tummy, with big stitch holes on either side of it. She put on her frilly nightie, fluffed the pillows and settled herself down for the arrival of Eddie Lane. Eddie was her neighbour, two years older than she, a widower with two grown-up children and two pet goats. She herself was fifty, fair, a little fat and doubtfully fertile. Eddie was getting new dentures. She anticipated what an improvement could do for his already perfect face.

There, right beside her on her bedside locker, were ten beautiful gall-stones wrapped in transparent plastic. If gall-stones could be judged as pearls, these would surely be prize-worthy.

Three-thirty on the dot! That familiar rap. In he came. Never empty handed. In his hand a plastic bag of what he knew would surprise and please her. He had only discovered these new yoghurt-flavoured peanuts of late, when he had been forced to look in the Health Food Shop for nettle tea for his born again naturalist sister. She who had smoked, drank and cavorted through the sixties now would not even drink tea. He placed the little plastic bag on the bedside locker.

'I've brought you a new sweetie. You'll love them.' Molly helped herself to a handful, and placed the bag in front of her bosom. 'Help yourself, Eddie, do have some.' Eddie eagerly popped his hand into the nearby bag, anticipating already the melting of the coating, and then the final crunch. He took two. He sucked and he sucked – no creamy melting. 'Strange,' he thought, and braced himself for the crunch.

The rest was a dental nightmare! He felt the crunch all right, felt it tearing through his jaws as he expertly broke his new dentures on two prime gall-stones. Molly was hysterical. It was all rather reminiscent of cannibalism, she thought. In the fray the yoghurt-coated peanuts and the gall-stones were mixed together on the floor. The following day Molly collected them all, and now was the proud owner of two hundred and ten gall-stones!

BRIDGET MAHER
Castletownroche
Co. Cork

Student's Triumph in Exam

The patient had recently come into Britain from the Far East. He was much the same age as the final year student who confronted him. He had had diarrhoea. 'Dysentry?' asked the final year student. 'I was told not to mention the names of diseases,' the patient returned in an apologetic tone. The student began to sweat into his best suit. This was the clinical 'quickie' in his Finals. He had ten minutes to make a diagnosis. He examined his patient for want of anything better to do. Abdomen, nothing. Rectum, nothing. Had he had blood-stained stools? 'Yes.' His patient, aware of his predicament, was delighted at a correct question.

The student looked for bacteriology findings but there were none. Time was running out. In despair he asked 'Are you taking any medication?' 'Prednisolone.' Light dawned. 'You've got ulcerative colitis.'

'My goodness,' said his patient as the professor appeared around the curtain. 'I wish I had come to you first. All those other doctors took weeks of testing and investigating before they found out what I had and you've found it out in five minutes.'

ELIZABETH SCOTT
Edinburgh

Hoax that failed:

Along the Canal

'Fine surgeons use fine catgut!' declared my surgical tutor, 'especially on the female abdomen. My God! what you're intending to use there looks more suitable for ligating the prepuce of a hippopotamus!'

Abdominal surgery requires a tough temperament, learning as you do from your mistakes. Just as well that I gave up surgery early in my career, for the alimentary tract has always caused me more problems than any other system – even before I became a student. It was, so to speak, in the bowels of the earth that I learned my first medical term 'duodenum', being the name given to a dim corridor running beneath the Royal Infirmary, Edinburgh, through the flexures of which those who have died in the wards above are taken on their last journey to the mortuary. The responsibility, in my day, was accorded to a porter named McDougal who, in his black uniform and peaked cap, carried the dourness of the Scots to extreme lengths, never having been heard to say anything other than 'Guid morning, nice day' to anyone, at any time, nor ever showing a trace of any emotion.

Working in bacteriology, I had made four friends in their final year who felt McDougal was an irresistible target for a practical joke. They decided, with Sister's co-operation, that Carstairs should be sewn into a winding sheet with an identification card attached at his head end. Then, McDougal would be summoned to take him down in the lift and along the duodenum, where, at a given signal, he would sit up on the trolley and groan. This would test McDougal's nerve and frighten him out of his skin, while we expressed our terror, and ran.

Once all was ready, Sister rang McDougal to report a male death on Ward Seven. Carstairs, a still white cotton cylinder just recognisable by the shoulders of a prop forward, was wheeled down the ward with due solemnity. The lift arrived. Its doors opened to reveal McDougal. 'Guid morning, nice day' he said, pulling the trolley into the lift. 'Do you mind if we come along with you?' asked Anderson, and we squeezed in either side of the supine Carstairs, and chatted naturally during the descent to the basement, carefully avoiding use of the code-word 'Murrayfield'.

Once we had reached the darkest part of the duodenum, the 'Sphincter of Oddi', we fell behind, finding it hard to refrain from giggling. Then, at the selected moment, Jamieson raised his voice, 'Shall I see you next week at Murrayfield?' at which good old Carstairs began tensing his recti abdominis, sitting up, letting out chilling cavernous groans. We almost spoiled the whole effect by exploding with laughter but managed to control it until it was stifled by McDougal's action as he took poor Carstairs by his rising shoulders, and brutually thrust him down shouting 'Get doon ye devil!' This, of course, made Carstairs panic but he was so tightly sewn in that he could barely flex his knees. Meanwhile McDougal, obviously thinking that the sooner he was in the cooler the better, had accelerated towards the place reserved now barely twenty yards away. The kinetic energy gained by the combined mass of McDougal hurrying and pushing the frantic figure of poor Carstairs crying for help inside his unyielding shroud was considerable, and we only just managed to stop further progress in front of the open door of the ice box. The joke had been on us.

Looking back I can see that, even if my own has served me well, the alimentary tract has always been a professional bugbear to me. For instance, in my final year I had difficulty learning chemical path, and went down to a place in England called Carshalton to work at it in the lab. I had only been there a couple of days when the pathologist told me that the casualty surgeons had heard there was a student working there, and would like me to help out as they were busy and short-staffed. 'But I'm not qualified,' I protested. 'Better go along and tell that to them,' he answered.

When I saw the casualty officers they said, 'Never mind that! You work in this room between us, and we'll let you have all the simple stuff, like cut fingers. If you have any problems, just call one of us.' As I had passed my surgery exams with flying colours I thought this practical experience would be a good form of tuition. So I agreed.

It turned out to be quite easy. I had dealt successfully with a grazed knee and a dog bite when in rushed an agitated mother, dragging her three-year-old daughter behind her. 'Quick, doctor! Do something!' she cried, 'Sheila's swallowed a threepenny bit!' Sheila looked fine, so, after a moment's reflexion, I thought a plain film would be a good idea to confirm the history, demonstrate the position of the coin, and so on. Half an hour later she returned with a wet film clearly indicating a heptagonal shadow. 'Ah! There it is', I said, stating the obvious, 'it's doing no harm and will be sure to pass through. So, keep a look out for it and come in again tomorrow.'

Next day, having removed a couple of splinters, and a f.b. from an eye, back came Sheila with her worried mother. 'No sign of it, doctor. No sign at all,' she complained. 'O.K. Let's have another film taken, it has probably gone.' But no, there it was in exactly the same place. So I said, 'Don't worry, she looks fine, and it's certain to be gone by tomorrow. Just take these notes and hand them to the clerk on your way out.' I was beginning to feel in control. The mother seemed to be developing confidence.

Next was an old man with a lump in the groin. 'Just drop your trousers behind the screen, and I'll come and have a look.' I was just going through the differential diagnosis in my mind: hernia? hydrocele? inguinal node? when suddenly the door burst open with force enough to knock the screen aside, exposing the senior citizen to about 200 people in the waiting hall outside as a female voice silenced everything, screaming: 'Call yourself a doctor? I think you're a disgrace! I'll see you struck off!' I rushed over to close the door, cover the old man's nakedness and deal with this abusive woman whom I now recognised as Sheila's mother, beside herself with righteous indigation. 'I'm sorry,' I said, 'but what is the nature of your complaint?' 'I'll tell you!' she shrieked. (I did not like to tell her that she could not fulfil her worst threat, to have me struck off, since I was not on the Register). 'There!' she cried, holding the record I had just given her in front of my face, 'just fancy making facetious remarks in the patient's notes when they are terribly worried and afraid!' And then she dropped the incriminating evidence on the floor and slammed the door behind her. I picked it up and read it, checking my first impulse to rush out and read to the assembled multitude in the hall outside what I had written, as they craned their necks to observe the offender, for what I had written was simply this: 'NO CHANGE. TCA TOMORROW'.

You may imagine that I had other thoughts about what I would be doing next day as I went in to see those who had recruited me. But, having steadied themselves from laughing, and declaring that it was the best thing they had heard that week, they closed in on me with serious faces and told me frankly that this was nothing compared to what I should have to face in the future. A tough skin was needed when dealing with the public. Next day it was a relief to be back in the calm atmosphere of the lab working on other peoples' bile salts.

M. KEITH THOMPSON
Croydon

Other misunderstandings easily arise when patients read their notes. For example, 'No change' on an X-ray report was interpreted as 'No chance', so the patient thought the outlook was hopeless.

The Surgeon's Sport

The anaesthetist sat at ease on his stool, his brogues highly polished beneath his gown.

'I miss going out with a gun to have a pot shot at the pheasants in the summer. Can't wait till the twelfth of August to come round. What about you, old chap?'

The surgeon, who was in the middle of a difficult hemicolectomy, swivelled a baleful eye.

'Why should I. I have surgery, the only blood sport with no close season.'

ELIZABETH SCOTT
Edinburgh

References

1 Burgess G.H.O. *The Curious World of Frank Buckland*. London: John Baker (1967)
2 Hawkins C. *Mishap or Malpractice?* Oxford: Blackwell Scientific Publications (1985)
3 Homer. *The Stay of Odysseus*, Ch XV (Translated by Rouse W.H.D.), p. 259. London: Thomas Nelson (1937)
4 de Montaigne Michel. *Familiar Medical Quotations*, (Ed. Strauss M.B.), p. 102. London: J. & A. Churchill (1968)
5 Hawkins C. Personal View: Diets. *British Medical Journal* (1970) **4**, 362
6 Aristophanes. *The Plutus*, Vol. III, No. 699. (Translated by Rogers B.B.) p. 427. London: Heinemann (1972)
7 Spiegl F. 'I'll Swear You're Mincing Your Words'. *The Independent*, 24 December (1987)
8 Aubrey's *Brief Lives* (Ed. Dick O.L.) p. 305. London: Secker and Warburg (1958)
9 Shaw H.W. 'Josh Billings': His Sayings. *Familiar Medical Quotations*, Ch 29. (Ed. Strauss M.B.) London: J. & A. Churchill (1968)
10 Osler Sir W. *Aphorisms for his Bedside Teachings and Writings* (Ed. Bean W.B.), 2nd edn. Springfield, Illinois: Charles C. Thomas (1961)
11 Plato. *The Republic*, Book III. No. 407 (Translated by Paul Shorey), p. 277. London: Heinemann (1969)
12 Marx K.F.H. Quoted by F.H. Garrison, *Bulletin of the New York Academy of Medicine* (1928) **4**,1001
13 Hawkins C.F. *Speaking and Writing in Medicine: The Art of Communication*. Springfield, Illinois: Charles C. Thomas (1967)
14 Anonymous. In England Now. *Lancet* (1959) ii, 1140
15 O'Dowd T.C. Five Years of Heartsink Patients in General Practice. *British Medical Journal* (1988) **297**,528–30
16 Gerrard T.J. & Riddell J.D. Difficult Patients. *British Medical Journal* (1988) **297**,530–2
17 Shaw H.W. 'Josh Billings': His Sayings. *Farmer's Alliminax*, March 1876. *Familiar Medical Quotations*, (Ed. Strauss M.B.), p. 230. London: J. & A. Churchill (1968)
18 Kipling R. A Doctor's work. An address to medical students at London's Middlesex Hospital *The Middlesex Hospital Journal* (1908) **xii**, 145–8
19 Hunt, Lord of Fawley. Doctors as Patients–Roles Reversed. *Transactions of the Medical Society of London* (1974) **90**, 1–19
20. Doyle C. *The Adventures of Sherlock Holmes: The Beryl Coronet*, p. 288. London: John Murray & Jonathan Cape (1974)

21 Colby F.M. The Colby Essays, 'Satire and Teeth' quoted in *The Writer and the Reader: A book of Literary Quotations* by Neil Ewart. Poole, Dorset: Blandford Press (1984) p 65

Men will confess to treason, murder, arson, false teeth, or a wig. How many of these will own up to a lack of humour?[21]

Index

abdominal pain
   due to home-made wine 63-4
   persistent 32-40, 90-4, 95-103,
      120-8
alcoholic intoxication
   due to home-made wine 63-4
   in infant 64-5
appendicitis, missed diagnosis
      95-102

belching
   effect on others 48-9, 120-8
   inflammable gases 47
belly ache *see* abdominal pain
borborygmi 21
bowel cancer, early diagnosis 77-84
bowels, British preoccupation with
      53-4
buccal smear, as test for bowel
      cancer 77-84

cholecystectomy 129
clothing, as bar to examination 24-7
communication, doctor-patient
      16-24, 49
constipation 53-4
corsets, dangers of 25-7
courage, seat of 1-4

defaecation
   routine of 53-4, 55-6
diagnoses
   correct 130
   incorrect 63-84
digestive system, reasoning behind
      design 4-6
dietary advice 42-6
doctor as patient 106-13
doctor-patient relationship 85-105

faeces
   analysis 60-2
   observation 59-60
food poisoning 20

furious bowel *see* irritable bowel

gall-stones, mistaken for peanuts
      128-9
general practice
   as battlefield 6-14
   guts needed for 1-4
girding the loins 1-4
gripe water, dangers of exceeding
      dose 64-5
guts, as site of fortitude 1-4

haemorrhoids 106-13
hashish swallowing, complications
      30-1
Heimlich manoeuvre 89
   adverse consequences 90-4
homeopath 116
hypochondriacs, dangers of crying
      'wolf' 85-94

in-service training 120-8
irritable bowel 32-41

King, Henry, unfortunate end 28-30
kordelbezoar 29-30

laparotomy 93
laxatives 54, 55-6

ME 87-8
Munchausen's syndrome, wrongly
      diagnosed 68-76
myalgic encephalomyelitis 87-8

obesity 21, 43, 44-5
objects swallowed 19, 28-31, 132-4
onomatopoeia and the guts 21-3,
      56-7
ovarian cyst, diagnosed as
      congestive cardiac failure 65-8
Oxford, Earl of, lapse 50

pain, descriptions of 20, 98

139